Critical Care Considerations of the Morbidly Obese

Guest Editors

MARILYN T. HAUPT, MD
MARY JANE REED, MD

CRITICAL CARE CLINICS

www.criticalcare.theclinics.com

Consulting Editor
RICHARD W. CARLSON, MD, PhD

October 2010 • Volume 26 • Number 4

SAUNDERS an imprint of ELSEVIER, Inc.

W.B. SAUNDERS COMPANY

A Division of Elsevier Inc.

Elsevier Inc. ● 1600 John F. Kennedy Blvd., ● Suite 1800 ● Philadelphia, Pennsylvania 19103-2899

http://www.theclinics.com

CRITICAL CARE CLINICS Volume 26, Number 4
October 2010 ISSN 0749-0704, ISBN-13: 978-1-4377-2437-0

Editor: Patrick Manley
Developmental Editor: Donald Mumford

Critical Care Clinics (ISSN: 0749-0704) is published quarterly by Elsevier Inc., 360 Park Avenue South, New York, NY 10010-1710. Months of issue are January, April, July, and October. Business and Editorial Offices: 1600 John F. Kennedy Blvd., Suite 1800, Philadelphia, PA 19103-2899. Customer Service Office: 6277 Sea Harbor Drive, Orlando, FL 32887-4800. Periodicals postage paid at New York, NY and additional mailing offices. Subscription prices are $179.00 per year for US individuals, $435.00 per year for US institution, $87.00 per year for US students and residents, $222.00 per year for Canadian individuals, $539.00 per year for Canadian institutions, $257.00 per year for international individuals, $539.00 per year for international institutions and $127.00 per year for Canadian and foreign students/residents. To receive student/resident rate, orders must be accompanied by name of affiliated institution, date of term, and the *signature* of program/residency coordinator on institution letterhead. Orders will be billed at individual rate until proof of status is received. Foreign air speed delivery is included in all *Clinics* subscription prices. All prices are subject to change without notice. POSTMASTER: Send address changes to *Critical Care Clinics*, Elsevier Periodicals Customer Service, 11830 Westline Industrial Drive, St. Louis, MO 63146. **Customer Service: 1-800-654-2452 (US). From outside of the US, call 1-314-447-8871. Fax: 1-314-447-8029. E-mail: journalscustomerservice-usa@elsevier.com (for print support) or journalsonlinesupport-usa@elsevier.com (for online support).**

Reprints. For copies of 100 or more of articles in this publication, please contact the Commercial Reprints Department, Elsevier Inc., 360 Park Avenue South, New York, NY 10010-1710. Tel.: 212-633-3813; Fax: 212-462-1935; E-mail: reprints@elsevier.com.

Critical Care Clinics is also published in Spanish by Editorial Inter-Medica, Junin 917, 1er A, 1113, Buenos Aires, Argentina.

Critical Care Clinics is covered in *MEDLINE/PubMed (Index Medicus), EMBASE/Excerpta Medica, Current Concepts/ Clinical Medicine, ISI/BIOMED, and Chemical Abstracts.*

Printed and bound in the United Kingdom

Transferred to Digital Print 2011

Contributors

CONSULTING EDITOR

RICHARD W. CARLSON, MD, PhD
Chairman Emeritus, Department of Medicine, Maricopa Medical Center and Director,
Medical Intensive Care Unit; Professor, University of Arizona College of Medicine;
and Professor, Department of Medicine, Mayo Graduate School of Medicine,
Phoenix, Arizona

GUEST EDITORS

MARILYN T. HAUPT, MD
Service Line Director, Pulmonary and Critical Care Medicine, Geisinger Health System;
Clinical Professor of Medicine, Temple University School of Medicine, Danville,
Pennsylvania

MARY JANE REED, MD, FACS, FASMBS, FCCM, FCCP
Associate, Departments of General Surgery and Critical Care Medicine, Geisinger
Medical Center; Clinical Professor of Medicine and Surgery, Temple University
Medical School, Danville, Pennsylvania

AUTHORS

KAREN ALLISON BAILEY, BSc, MD, FRCSC
Pediatric General Surgery, Co-director of Pediatric Trauma Program, McMaster
Children's Hospital; Assistant Professor, McMaster University, Hamilton,
Ontario, Canada

DENNIS E. AMUNDSON, DO, MS, FCCM
Department of Pulmonary/Critical Care Medicine, Naval Medical Center San Diego,
San Diego, California

DOYLE D. ASHBURN, DO
Department of Critical Care Medicine, Geisinger Medical Center, Danville, Pennsylvania

MARIE R. BALDISSERI, MD, FCCM
Associate Professor, Department of Critical Care Medicine, University of Pittsburgh
Medical Center, Pittsburgh, Pennsylvania

PETER N. BENOTTI, MD, FACS
Residency Program Director, Department of Surgery, St Francis Medical Center, Trenton,
New Jersey

ION D. BUCALOIU, MD
Associate, Department of Nephrology, Geisinger Medical Center, Danville, Pennsylvania

MICHELE CHAMBERLAIN, BSN, RN, CBN
Bariatric and Minimally Invasive Nurse Coordinator, Bariatric Surgery Department, Geisinger Medical Center, Danville, Pennsylvania

MICHAEL CLARK, MD
Associate, Department of Otolaryngology, Geisinger Medical Center, Danville, Pennsylvania

MITCHELL K. CRAFT, DO
Critical Care Medicine Fellow, Division of Critical Care Medicine, Geisinger Medical Center, Danville, Pennsylvania

ANGELA DEANTONIO, MD, FCCP
Department of Critical Care Medicine, Geisinger Wyoming Valley Medical Center, Wilkes-Barre, Pennsylvania

WILLIAM DIFILIPPO, MD
Associate, Department of Nephrology, Geisinger Medical Center, Danville, Pennsylvania

SVETOLIK DJURKOVIC, MD
Department of Medicine, Inova Health System Critical Care Medicine, Falls Church, Virginia

JON GABRIELSEN, MD, FACS, FASMBS
Associate, Department of Bariatric Surgery, Geisinger Medical Center, Danville, Pennsylvania

JAMES GEILING, MD, FACP, FCCM
Chief, Medical Service, Veterans Affairs Medical Center, White River Junction, Vermont; Professor of Medicine, New England Center for Emergency Preparedness, Dartmouth Medical School, Hanover, New Hampshire

SCOTT GREENE, DO
Associate, Department of Otolaryngology, Geisinger Medical Center, Danville, Pennsylvania

MARGARET D. LARKINS-PETTIGREW, MD, MEd, MPPM
Assistant Professor, Department of Obstetrics, Gynecology and Reproductive Sciences, MacDonald Women's, Case Western University Medical Center, Cleveland, Ohio

WILLIAM A. LODER, MD
Departments of Anesthesiology and Critical Care Medicine, Geisinger Medical Center, Danville, Pennsylvania

GREGORY N. MATWIYOFF, MD
Pulmonary Critical Care and Sleep Medicine, Naval Medical Center San Diego, San Diego, California

CHARLES J. MEDICO, PharmD, BCPS
Board Certified Pharmacotherapy Specialist, Division of System Therapeutics and Critical Care Medicine, Geisinger Medical Center, Danville, Pennsylvania; Adjunct Assistant Professor, Department of Pharmacy Practice, Wilkes University Nesbitt School of Pharmacy, Wilkes-Barre, Pennsylvania; Pharmacy Clinical Coordinator, System Therapeutics, Geisinger Medical Center, Danville, Pennsylvania

EVAN NORFOLK, MD
Associate, Department of Nephrology, Geisinger Medical Center, Danville, Pennsylvania

MICHELLE OLSON, MD, FACS, FASCRS
Associate, Department of General Surgery, Geisinger Medical Center; Clinical Professor of Surgery, Temple Medical School, Danville, Pennsylvania

ROBERT M. PERKINS, MD
Associate, Department of Nephrology, Geisinger Medical Center; Clinical Investigator, Biostatistics Research and Data Core, Henry Hood Center for Health Research, Danville, Pennsylvania

CHRIS POHL, MD
Associate, Department of Interventional Radiology, Geisinger Medical Center, Danville, Pennsylvania

OMAR RAHMAN, MD
Medical Director, Adult Intensive Care/Shock Trauma Unit, Geisinger Medical Center; Associate, Department of Critical Care Medicine, Geisinger Medical Center, Danville, Pennsylvania

NAEEM RAZA, MD
Fellow, Department of Gastroenterology and Nutrition, Geisinger Medical Center, Pennsylvania

MARY JANE REED, MD, FACS, FASMBS, FCCM, FCCP
Associate, Departments of General Surgery and Critical Care Medicine, Geisinger Medical Center; Clinical Professor of Medicine and Surgery, Temple University Medical School, Danville, Pennsylvania

CHRISTOPHER D. STILL, DO, FACN, FACP
Associate, Department of Gastroenterology and Nutrition; Medical Director, Center for Nutrition and Weight Management; Director, Geisinger Obesity Institute; Geisinger Health System, Pennsylvania

ROBERT STRONY, DO
Associate, Department of Emergency Medicine, Geisinger Medical Center, Danville, Pennsylvania

CHRISTINE C. TOEVS, MD, FACS, FCCM
Roanoke, Virginia

PATRICK WALSH, DO, FCCP
Intensivist, Division of Critical Care Medicine, Geisinger Medical Center, Danville, Pennsylvania; Adjunct Assistant Professor, Temple University School of Medicine, Philadelphia, Pennsylvania

LAUREL WILLIS, PA-C
Physician Assistant, Department of Critical Care Medicine, Geisinger Medical Center, Danville, Pennsylvania

TAHER YAHYA, MD
Associate, Department of Nephrology, Geisinger Medical Center, Danville, Pennsylvania

Contents

examines the literature pertinent to AKI in critically ill MO patients. After a concise review of the available epidemiologic data regarding the incidence of acute renal injury in MO individuals, the authors review the limitations and available tools for estimation of renal function in the MO population (with emphasis on the critical illness). Also described are several specific types of renal injury previously described in this population that are applicable to the critical care setting. Lastly, the authors review some of the challenges and limitations in providing renal support to critically ill MO individuals, and identify potential areas for future research in this population.

Several significant changes occur in the gastrointestinal system with obesity that can effect management in critical illness. This population is at risk for gastroesophageal reflux disease (GERD), abdominal compartment syndrome, nonalcoholic fatty liver disease (NAFLD), and an increased incidence of cholelithiasis. It is important for critical care providers to be aware of these potential complicating factors.

A growing body of literature suggests multifaceted alterations to the immune function in obese patients compared with a lean cohort. Although treatment in the intensive care unit has an associated risk of infectious complications, which, if any, of these immunologic alterations are causal is unclear. Obesity clearly causes abundant alterations to the immune system. Overall, the aggregate effect seems to be chronic activation of inflammatory mediators.

Obesity is associated with significant alterations in endocrine function. An association with type 2 diabetes mellitus and dyslipidemia has been well documented. This article highlights the complexities of treating endocrine system disorders in obese patients.

Venous thromboembolic disease continues to be a major source of morbidity and mortality, with obese patients who are critically ill presenting some of the most at-risk patients. As the literature evolves, it has become clear that there is a complex relationship between obesity and thrombosis and atherogenesis. It is true that many of these conditions are reversible with weight loss; however, obesity remains on the rise. Management of obese patients must incorporate and consider these intricate changes in an attempt to improve patient outcomes.

disease, skin disorders such as intertrigo and cellulitis, and urinary incontinence. Thus, patients exposed to a variety of disasters not only are increasingly overweight but also have an associated number of coexistent medical conditions that require increased support with medical devices and medications. This article focuses on management of the morbidly obese patients during disasters.

The critically ill pregnant patient poses a unique challenge to the clinician, requiring a thorough understanding of normal and abnormal maternal and fetal physiology associated with pregnancy. The morbidly obese patient presents even greater challenges to the clinician, and morbidity and mortality are proportionately increased. Because increased numbers of obese pregnant women are now admitted to intensive care units, practitioners must be aware of the physiology associated with both pregnancy and obesity. A multidisciplinary approach is imperative to prevent both maternal and fetal morbidity and mortality for these very complex patients, especially when they are admitted to the ICU with critical illness.

THE CLINICS ARE NOW AVAILABLE ONLINE!

Access your subscription at:
www.theclinics.com

Preface

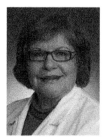 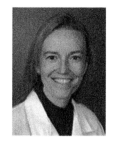

Marilyn T. Haupt, MD   Mary Jane Reed, MD, FACS,
                             FASMBS, FCCM, FCCP
              Guest Editors

As critical care practitioners, we have seen our ICU transformed over the last 20 years from a facility challenged with the care of an occasional morbidly obese patient to one that cares for multiple morbidly obese patients on a daily basis. Nevertheless, our approach to the management continues to be primarily empiric and without guidance from clinical research directed toward this population of patients. Although research is evolving in this area, large gaps in knowledge persist. Optimal dosing, for example, is unknown for many drugs, including those that may be lifesaving. Although a modest body of literature exists on antibiotic dosing in the obese, the studies addressing dosing of cardiac medications in these patients are infrequent and sporadic. Controversy continues to persist over whether a calorie-restricted diet is safe or beneficial in the critically ill obese patient.

To address these care challenges, we enthusiastically embraced the opportunity to organize this collection of articles addressing the care of the critically ill obese and morbidly obese patient. Practitioners and clinical researchers with experience and interest have authored these articles, providing scientific backup whenever possible as well as wisdom and common sense that derives from years of practice. We hope that clinicians will find useful applications of this knowledge base and that clinical researchers will recognize areas requiring investigation.

Crit Care Clin 26 (2010) xiii–xiv
doi:10.1016/j.ccc.2010.09.005   **criticalcare.theclinics.com**

Marilyn T. Haupt, MD
Pulmonary and Critical Care Medicine
Geisinger Health System
Temple University School of Medicine
100 North Academy Avenue
Mail Code: 20-37
Danville, PA 17822, USA

Mary Jane Reed, MD, FACS, FASMBS, FCCM, FCCP
Departments of General Surgery and Critical Care Medicine
Geisinger Medical Center
Temple University Medical School
100 North Academy Avenue
Mail Code: 20-37
Danville, PA 17822, USA

E-mail addresses:
mthaupt@geisinger.edu (M.T. Haupt)
mreed@geisinger.edu (M.J. Reed)

The Obesity Paradox

Dennis E. Amundson, DO, MS, FCCS[a],*, Svetolik Djurkovic, MD[b],
Gregory N. Matwiyoff, MD[c]

KEYWORDS

• Obesity • Obesity paradox • Consequences of obesity

THE OBESITY PARADOX

The term "obesity paradox" refers to the observations that, although obesity is a major risk factor in the development of cardiovascular and peripheral vascular disease, when acute cardiovascular decompensation occurs, for example, in myocardial infarction or congestive heart failure, obese patients may have a survival benefit.[1] In addition, it has been suggested that obese patients tend to fare better after certain surgical procedures, such as coronary artery bypass surgery.[2–4] Moreover, it appears that obese men with chronic hypertensive heart disease live longer than men of normal weight.

Major hypotheses for this apparent survival effect include:

1. Obese patients may have better and more aggressive medical care and enhanced observation than normal-weight populations.
2. Obese patients tend to be on more, and perhaps better, cardioprotective medical therapy than other groups of patients.
3. Obese patients tend to be younger at the time of the acute cardiovascular event, which may confer an age benefit.
4. Some experts claim the sample size of the existing studies on obesity is still too small or too indecisive to make such determinations.[5]
5. Other investigators suggest the way we measure obesity is unsatisfactory and may explain some of the paradoxic results seen. Specifically, using gross weight and the

Conflict of interest: None.
Financial support: None.
The views expressed in this article are those of the authors and do not reflect the official policy or position of the Department of the Navy, Department of Defense, or the United States Government.
[a] Department of Pulmonary/Critical Care Medicine, Naval Medical Center San Diego, San Diego, CA, USA
[b] Department of Medicine, Inova Health System Critical Care Medicine, 3300 Gallows Road, Falls Church, VA 22042-3300, USA
[c] Pulmonary Critical Care and Sleep Medicine, Naval Medical Center San Diego, San Diego, CA, USA
* Corresponding author.
E-mail address: dennis.amundson@med.navy.mil

body mass index (BMI) may not accurately reflect the risk of complications in all obese individuals.[6]

These factors may lead to the false impression that obesity confers some survival advantage with acute cardiovascular stress and in some chronic conditions. However, mounting evidence shows that obesity alone may confer a survival benefit independent of age, medical care, or therapy. Perhaps the definition of obesity needs to be revisited, and it is also possible that "all fat is not equal."

The following questions can be posed:

1. Does the literature support a salutary effect of obesity on acute cardiovascular events and improvement in chronic disease-state mortality?
2. If it is true that all fat is not the same, what would be the mechanistic or physiologic changes in these individuals that could confer such effect?
3. Conversely, Might the presence of a normal or reduced BMI be detrimental in someone with an acute cardiovascular event?

The Obesity Epidemic

Approximately 65% of United States citizens can be classified as overweight and 30% are frankly obese.[7] The prevalence differs by age, sex, and ethnicity, but increases are seen in all demographic sectors. Obesity is considered epidemic in the United States, as well as in the world in general, and it is an increasingly major health hazard in many developing nations.[8] Obesity is clearly associated with the development of some common chronic conditions, and obese individuals have between 50% and 100% increase in the chance of early death when compared with people of normal weight.

However, not all fat is created equal. For years, we have known that mutations in the melanocortin-4 receptor gene contribute to a variety of phenotypes in the obese individual. These phenotypes lead to a variety of metabolic responses, which may vary.[9] Different gene mutations may lead to completely different "obesity syndromes," with potentially different risks for sequelae. Moreover, weight distribution seems to be a factor in risk stratification, with waist-to-hip ratios apparently being important in determining the phenotype and subsequent effects.[6]

At present, the conventional way to categorize obesity is by the body mass index (BMI):

$$BMI = weight\ (kg)/[height\ (m)^2]$$
$$BMI = weight\ in\ pounds/(height\ in\ inches)^2$$

BMI (kg/m^2) categories are:
BMI <18.5 = underweight
BMI 18.5–24.9 = normal weight
BMI 25–29.9 = overweight
BMI >30 = obese
BMI >40 (or $>35\ kg/m^2$ + comorbidity) = morbid ("clinically severe") obesity
BMI >50 = "super-obesity"

Pathophysiology of Obesity

Clinical obesity is a syndrome involving both weight and metabolic changes, and is influenced by both genetic and environmental factors. Both aspects can participate in the pathology associated with obesity. The specific factors can be categorized into weight-related, physiologic, and proinflammatory. All may participate in the response to acute stressors. See **Box 1.**

Box 1
Overview of pathophysiologic effects of obesity

Weight-Related Changes

    Degenerative joint disease

    Dermal pressure changes

    Restrictive pulmonary physiology

    Increased intra-abdominal pressure effects

    Mobility limitations

Physiologic Changes

    Hyperkinetic systemic circulation

    Myocardial hypertrophy

    Elevated systemic pressure

    Diastolic dysfunction

    Increased circulating blood volume

    Metabolic syndrome

Proinflammatory Phenotypic Changes

    Vascular intimal atherosclerotic changes

    Prothrombotic state with:

        Increased fibrinogen

        Decreased fibrinolysis

        Increased antithrombin-III levels

        Increased plasmin activator inhibitor levels

        Increased blood viscosity

Obesity and Cancer

In terms of cancer development, it seems clear from both animal studies and human epidemiologic data that leaner individuals have less cancer risk. Animal studies suggest that animals fed at 60% of controls have fewer cancers.[10] The relationship is subtle, however, and no physiologic mechanism can be found to explain these observations. Obesity has been linked to 20% of all cancer deaths in women and 14% in men.[11]

How does obesity contribute to increased risk of cancer?

    Hyperinsulinemia. The proposed mechanism is via insulin-like growth factor (IGF) that starts a signaling cascade resulting in:
        Increased cell division
        Interruption in cell death
    Increased estradiol. Adipose tissue increases conversion of androgenic precursors to estradiol through increased aromatase activity in adipose tissue. Estrogens have been shown to be mitogenic and mutagenic, inducing direct or indirect free radical mediated DNA damage. In endometrial cancer, for instance, estradiol increases endometrial cell proliferation, inhibits apoptosis, and stimulates IGF-1.

Increased levels of circulating leptin
Increased adipose tissue hypoxia
Increased system inflammation/elevated C-reactive protein

The study by Calle and colleagues[10] in 2003 of 900,000 United States adults demonstrated that the incidence of many cancers (esophagus, colon, rectal, liver, gallbladder, pancreas, kidney, non-Hodgkin, lymphoma, melanoma) is directly related to BMI. In addition, the mortality rate is higher in certain malignancies (stomach, prostate, breast, uterus, cervix, ovary) in the overweight population. The BMI seems to linearly follow cancer mortality. In summary, in the case of malignancy, it appears that obesity both increases the risk of developing cancer and increases the risk of death in those who develop cancer. Thus, the literature does not support a protective effect of obesity in malignancy.

Obesity and Hypertension

Substantial evidence from epidemiologic data supports a link between obesity and hypertension. In addition, numerous pathophysiological mechanisms link obesity and hypertension. Obesity raises blood pressure by increasing renal tubular reabsorption, impairing pressure natriuresis, causing volume expansion due to activation of the sympathetic nervous system and the renin-angiotensin system, and by physical compression of the kidneys, especially when visceral obesity is present. The mechanisms of sympathetic nervous system activation in obesity may be caused, in part, by hyperleptinemia and hyperinsulinemia.[12] Leptin is a cytokine derived from the adipocytes and released into the bloodstream. In obese humans, serum leptin levels are increased and correlate with the individual's BMI and blood pressure. Leptin induces endothelin-1 (ET-1), a potent vasoconstrictor and mitogen, as well as endothelin type A receptor expression, on vascular smooth muscle cells.[13,14] In rats, chronic infusion of leptin to achieve serum leptin levels comparable to those observed in obese individuals induced hypertension. Hyperinsulinemia can contribute to the development of hypertension by activating the sympathetic nervous system, by causing sodium retention, and by stimulation of secretion of ET-1 from vascular endothelium.[15] The impact of obesity on mortality in patients with hypertension, however, is less clear. Studies addressing this question showed conflicting results. Stamler and colleagues[16] demonstrated that lean hypertensive patients (BMI <22) have increased 8-year mortality when compared with overweight hypertensives. Nevertheless, they were able to explain this excess in mortality with differences in comorbidities and lifestyle between the 2 groups as contributing to both leanness and risk of death. Among men, smokers and nonsmokers had higher death rates at a low BMI. Deaths related to lifestyle factors, such as smoking and alcohol intake, contributed to the excess risk, particularly among lean persons with hypertension.[16] In 800 hypertensive patients, overall mortality and cardiovascular and noncardiovascular events were highest in the patients at the leanest BMI quintile. The association between BMI and cardiovascular end points was U-shaped, whereas noncardiovascular mortality decreased with increasing BMI. The BMI level with the lowest risk was 28 to 29 kg/m^2 for overall mortality, 26 to 27 kg/m^2 for cardiovascular mortality, and 31 to 32 kg/m^2 for noncardiovascular mortality. The study of low-dose antihypertensive therapy in the elderly showed similar results. There was no statistically significant relation of death or stroke with BMI in the placebo group, and there was a U-shaped relation in the treatment group. These results persisted after controlling for multiple covariates. The lowest probability of death for men was associated with a BMI of 26.0 and for women with a BMI of 29.6.[17] The analysis of the data of 22,576 patients from the International Verapamil SR-Trandolapril Study (INVEST) cohort showed an approximately 30% lower 2-year mortality in overweight and obese patients compared with the normal-weight group. In addition, patients with BMIs of 30 to 35 kg/m^2 had the lowest mortality, despite having smaller blood pressure reduction compared with patients of normal weight at 24 months.[18] The answer to the question of whether obese patients with hypertension fare better is not straightforward. There may be several possible biases that could explain this apparent survival advantage which may be difficult to account for, such as socioeconomic status, smoking, medical care received, and other comorbid conditions. Several studies, for example, have shown that obese hypertensive patients in trials are younger than nonobese patients. Not only would younger age give them an advantage in terms of survival, but they would also constitute a different cohort compared with the older patients. Patients who lose weight involuntarily are likely to have severe underlying diseases, and their life expectancy might be shorter, in contrast to patients who lose weight intentionally with lifestyle modifications, who have better outcomes.[19] The "fit fat" effect assumes that only fit obese patients survive and have no exclusion criteria to be included in the studies. In patients who gain weight at an older age, several competing risk factors might affect outcome before the effects of obesity become manifest.

On the other hand, obesity might confer protection by various mechanisms involved in inflammatory and hormonal homeostasis. Obese patients may have higher energy reserve, which could be especially important during acute disease. The effects of obesity on pharmacokinetics also are not well understood. Several investigators speculate that obese patients might tolerate higher doses of renin-angiotensin inhibition. At present, a body of literature suggests a survival benefit to obesity in chronic hypertension.

Obesity and Chronic Kidney Disease

In addition to the link between obesity and diabetes and hypertension, obesity plays an independent role in the development of renal disease. Obesity leads to glomerular hyperfiltration, increased urinary albumin loss, and a progressive loss of renal function associated with a focal segmental glomerulosclerosis. This situation may be present not only in subjects with previously manifest renal disease but also in otherwise healthy subjects. These renal changes may be related to insulin resistance and/or hyperleptinemia, but may also be mediated by a state of low-grade inflammation induced by obesity.[20]

Data from the Framingham cohort show that obesity is associated with an increased risk of developing stage 3 chronic kidney disease (CKD) over nearly 20 years of follow-up. This association was no longer observed after adjustment for cardiovascular disease (CVD) risk factors, suggesting the association of obesity with chronic renal insufficiency may be mediated by CVD risk factors.[21] Madero and colleagues, in observing 1759 CKD patients, found a survival advantage at later stage III CKD and higher, and importantly, advantage seemed to be independent of other risk factors. However, once end-stage renal disease (ESRD) develops, obese patients seem to have survival benefit as compared with the lean subjects. In patients with ESRD on hemodialysis, lower BMI is consistently found to be a strong predictor of an elevated mortality in numerous studies.[22–28] Furthermore, a higher BMI in the mild-to-moderate range is generally associated with a decrease in mortality risk in patients with ESRD. Most studies have shown that the inverse association between BMI and mortality in patients with ESRD on both hemodialysis and peritoneal dialysis is independent of serum albumin and other markers of nutritional status. Only a few small studies show no benefit or increased risk of mortality with increased BMI in patients on hemodialysis.[29,30] Most,[31–39] but not all,[40,41] studies show better survival with increased BMI in patients on peritoneal dialysis. The possible explanations of this survival benefit with increasing BMI in patients with ESRD were summarized in a review by Kalantar-Zadeh and colleagues.[42]

More stable hemodynamic status in obese patients
Overweight and obese patients tend to have higher systemic blood pressure values and may better tolerate load-reducing agents, such as angiotensin-converting enzyme inhibitors.

Tumor necrosis factor-α receptors in obesity
Adipose tissue produces soluble tumor necrosis factor (TNF)-α receptors, which result in higher circulating concentrations of receptors in obese subjects. Soluble TNF-α receptors may play a cardioprotective role because they neutralize the adverse biologic effects of TNF-α and may contribute to progressive cardiac injury through their proapoptotic and negative inotropic effects.

Neurohormonal alterations in obesity
Sympathetic and renin-angiotensin activities are associated with a poor prognosis in fluid overload states. Sympathetic and renin-angiotensin responses during exercise in obese patients are blunted compared with lean subjects.

Endotoxin-lipoprotein hypothesis
Greater lipopolysaccharide (LPS) concentrations have been shown in persons with fluid overload than in the general population. Obese dialysis patients whose serum cholesterol concentrations generally tend to be higher could better neutralize circulating LPS, and therefore decrease inflammation and subsequent atherosclerosis.

Malnutrition-inflammation complex syndrome
If overweight patients with an increase in adipose tissue develop a deficiency in energy or protein intake, they would be less likely to develop frank protein-energy malnutrition. Underweight patients with ESRD would more likely become ill and would recover more slowly from illness compared with patients who have normal weight or who are overweight.

Reverse causation
Reverse causation is a known possible source of bias. Comorbid states may lead to wasting and also to a higher rate of mortality. Obesity would be barely a marker of better health.

Survival bias
The majority of patients with CKD die before requiring dialysis. Dialysis patients might therefore be "the fittest." Obese patients in this subgroup would thus not represent the selected subgroup, and their survival advantage would not be generalizable.

Time discrepancies among competitive risk factors
Obese patients with ESRD often have numerous comorbidities and may die from "competing" comorbidities before the consequences of the obesity could manifest.

OBESITY AND CARDIOVASCULAR DISEASE

As noted previously, obesity seems to be clearly associated with an increased risk of untoward cardiovascular disease and cardiovascular outcomes. Nonetheless, some data are accruing that suggest improved outcomes in chronic heart failure. In 2005, Curtis and colleagues[1] looked at data from more than 7000 heart failure patients enrolled in a National Heart, Blood, and Lung Institute digitalis study; they evaluated all-cause mortality categorized by BMI and found a near-linear decrease in all-cause mortality associated with increasing BMI. In 2006, Romero-Corral and colleagues[4] performed a meta-analysis of all available studies looking at body weight and cardiovascular mortality, as well as BMI associations; they, too, found low BMI to be associated with an increase in mortality and an increase in recurrent cardiovascular events. The association of higher BMIs with improved outcomes was conflicted over the 40 studies reviewed, but obesity was an independent, positive survival factor when followed over an average of 3.8 years.[4] Most important, the "massively obese" population did appear to have more cardiovascular deaths, but overall mortality remained slightly less than for the normal-weight population. This study suggested that overweight and mild-to-moderate obesity conferred survival advantage over normal-weight individuals after all confounders were assessed.[4]

Obesity and Acute Stressors

Sepsis and obesity

Both sepsis incidence and septic mortality continue to increase throughout the world, as does the incidence of obesity in the world population. Therefore, increasingly, the obese patient population uses critical care resources and increasingly is admitted for severe sepsis or septic shock. Is there an association between the septic milieu and the biologic/metabolic effects of obesity?

Pathophysiologically, sepsis mediates most of its detrimental effects by an alteration of the host immune system. This inflammatory response engenders a complex multifaceted event that frequently leads to organ dysfunction and widespread oxygen debt. Many times the response is associated with "multiple organ dysfunction syndrome" and its attendant high mortality and costly resource use. Some of the host responses include cellular activation, intracellular cytokine response/release, inflammatory cascade initiation, endovascular inflammation, and macro- and microvascular coagulation activation via the extrinsic pathway.[43]

As noted previously, obesity confers an alteration in the inflammatory response that tends to be proinflammatory and has local weight effects that hinder normal mucosal, humoral, and cellular responses. In addition, organ effects of obesity, such as seen in the cardiovascular system or with the diabetic state, could be expected to abrogate a normal homeostatic response to a septic stressor. In addition, both intracellular cytokines and activation of bioactive polypeptides found in adipose tissue have been shown to be linked to sepsis. These polypeptides, or adipokines, may participate in the inflammatory host response (**Box 2**).[43]

Given all the potential inflammatory mediators involved in the obesity-sepsis relationship, it would seem the proinflammatory obesity phenotype may be detrimental in a septic state. However, human data on the obesity-sepsis interaction are lacking. It does appear that obese patients fare worse in general trauma, postoperatively, and in medical intensive care units (ICUs).[46–50] Most of these small observational studies show an increase in ICU days, wound complications, and infections. A few studies have suggested there is an increase in mortality in the obese ICU patient.[51] It is interesting that most of these prior studies also illustrated that the low BMI patient had elevated morbidity and mortality.

Akinnusi and colleagues[52] recently completed a meta-analysis of 62,045 critical care patients. Although criticized for some of the analysis assumptions, they also

---

Box 2
Adipokines

Leptin

    Has a hypothalamic action on pre-melanocortin and insulin

    Elevated levels are found in sepsis and may be predictive of severity of sepsis[44]

Adiponectin

    Anti-inflammatory protein that regulates insulin sensitivity. May be protective for endothelial dysfunction. Tends to decrease in sepsis that may follow severity. May be modulated by nuclear factor-(kappa) B

    kappa-B inversely correlates with body fat[45]

Resistin

    Proinflammatory protein produced by white blood cells, involved in insulin resistance. High levels may correlate with increased sepsis severity. Also, levels may indicate a prolonged inflammatory state[46]

---

demonstrate an overall increase in morbidity, but not in mortality, in obese ICU patients, many of whom were septic.

In summary, the best available evidence currently suggests that morbidity, ICU duration, ICU complications, and ICU cost may be increased in the obese patient who has sepsis. However, a mortality increase has not been clearly identified, and no obesity paradox can be clearly seen in this population. More work is needed to demonstrate a clear outcome difference in the septic obese patient.

Obesity and Postoperative Response

Although controversial, several older studies (and conventional wisdom) suggest an increase in postoperative complications in the obese surgical patient. Most of these complications, though, are usually minor skin/wound infections and minor difficulties in local care. A clear increased risk of postoperative death has not been found in the obese. The studies on this are small in number and are usually retrospective, single-institution, population reviews. Recently, a large-scale database (American College of Surgeons, National Surgical Quality Improvement Program) study was performed; more than 150,000 procedures were analyzed during the period of 2005 to 2006, and data from 118,707 cases were abstracted for weight variables and outcomes,[49] The usual measures to ensure a validation of a large database sample were performed, and the variables included outcomes process of care, cost, time, and adverse events (10 groups). BMI classes were compared and regression analysis was performed.[49] Results of the analysis were particularly robust, and the cases did include laparoscopic procedures.[49] Some disparity was seen with procedure, age, and sex in the obese, but overall a broad, well-represented spectrum was obtained and analyzed.[49] One significant issue was that underweight patients seemed to undergo longer and more complex procedures than any other class.[49]

As noted in this study and in some prior smaller studies, underweight patients had a significantly higher 30-day mortality (5%) than the other classes. In the overweight class, postoperative mortality (1.2%) was less than in the normal-weight class (1.8%); however, it increased by overweight category (1.0%–1.3%). The overall odds ratio and 95% confidence interval (CI) for mortality was 2.80 and 2.30 to 3.38, respectively. The graphical regression curve demonstrated the reverse J-shaped relationship found in other studies, demonstrating the obesity paradox. These data, although somewhat hampered by the difficulty in defining BMI as a single variable, are the largest and best sources of information available on the postoperative patient, and clearly support an obesity paradox with nonbariatric surgical procedures.[53]

Using the same database, vascular procedures in 7500 patients were similarly examined, although the risk factors of diabetes and hypertension were higher in the obese categories.[54] The mortality curve showed a J-shape over normal-weight individuals. This finding is also supported by information from the Scottish Coronary Revascular Registry for Percutaneous Revascularization. Over a 9-year period (1997–2008), this study showed individuals with BMI 27.5 or more and less than 30 had reduced 5-year death rates (hazard ratio [HR] 0.59, 95% CI 0.39–0.90. $P \leq .014$). These data on improved postoperative survival in the moderately obese need to be recognized.

Postcoronary revascularization risk has been assessed. A meta-analysis of the existing databases was performed, which addressed both short-term (30-day) and long-term (5-year) all-cause mortality.[55] Both coronary artery bypass grafting and percutaneous procedures were analyzed, with more than 20 studies reviewed. The summary data found an improved early all-cause mortality in the overweight/obese in attendance over the observation time, and also showed a J-shape for cure duration and mortality with a higher degree of obesity. This trend was observed in both preventative and operative revascularization procedures.

Obesity in Acute Heart Failure

That obesity is a risk factor for all-cause and cardiovascular mortality, myocardial infarction, and heart failure is indisputable.[56,57] However, an emerging body of literature suggests that patients who are overweight or obese with established cardiovascular disease have a reduced risk of adverse outcomes, including mortality.[58]

By far the largest and strongest body of literature supporting an inverse relationship between BMI and adverse outcomes in cardiovascular disease is found in studies in patients with heart failure.[58–60] The recognition that a paradoxic relationship between body weight and adverse outcomes is not new. Between 1983 and 1999, Horwich and colleagues[61] observed that among approximately 1200 patients with heart failure who were referred for heart transplant, those who were obese (BMI >31) had a significant survival benefit at 2 years.

The association between increasing body weight and reduction in adverse cardiovascular outcome was further demonstrated in studies involving patients with stable heart failure and acute decompensated heart failure, as well as in a recent meta-analysis that included more than 28,000 patients with congestive heart failure.[59]

Analysis of data from the Digitalis Investigation Group (DIG) by Curtis and colleagues[62] demonstrated that in 7767 patients who were categorized based on BMI and after controlling for more than 20 variables, all-cause mortality rates decreased in a linear manner with increasing BMI. All-cause mortality ranged from 45% in the underweight group with BMI lass than 18.5 to 28.4% in the obese group (BMI >30), with a P value of less than .001. The investigators concluded that in patients with stable heart failure, a higher BMI is independently associated with a lower risk of death and death from worsening heart failure.

Fonarow and colleagues[60] evaluated the mortality risk in decompensated heart failure in a retrospective review of 108,927 patients who had been admitted with the diagnosis of heart failure from 2001 through 2004. After adjustment for age, gender, blood pressure, heart rate, dyspnea, blood urea nitrogen, creatinine, and sodium, in-hospital mortality decreased with successively higher BMI quartiles, such that for every 5-unit increase in BMI, the odds of risk-adjusted mortality were reduced by 10% (95% CI 0.88–0.93 $P<.0001$).

More recently, Oreopoulos and colleagues[59] conducted a meta-analysis including 9 observational studies with 28,209 patients. These investigators found that in patients classified as overweight (BMI 25–29) and obese (BMI >30), there was a reduction in all-cause mortality, and in a risk-adjusted sensitivity analysis, being overweight (adjusted HR 0.93, 95% CI 0.89–0.97) or obese (adjusted HR 0.88, 95% CI 0.83–0.93) was protective against mortality.

A robust body of literature associating elevated BMI with reduced adverse outcomes also exists in patients with coronary disease. Mehta and colleagues,[63] in a meta-analysis including 40 cohort studies with over 250,000 patients with coronary artery disease, demonstrated an inverse association between increasing BMI and mortality. This association has been further demonstrated in patients undergoing percutaneous coronary intervention, with obese patients demonstrating a lower incidence of major hospital complications such as bleeding, myocardial infarction, and cardiac death.[64,65]

Uretsky and colleagues[19] reported that in 22,576 patients with hypertension and coronary artery disease, a significant reduction in the primary outcome was found, including occurrence of death, nonfatal myocardial infarction, or nonfatal stroke in patients defined as overweight (BMI 25–29) (HR 0.77, 95% CI 0.7–0.86, $P<.001$), class I obesity (BMI 30–35) (HR 0.68, 95% CI 0.59–0.78, $P<.001$), and class II obesity (BMI >35) (adjusted HR 0.76, 95% CI 0.65–0.88), with class I obesity patients having the lowest risk of primary outcome.

An inverse relationship between infarct size and obesity (BMI >30) was reported in a study using contrast-enhanced magnetic resonance imaging to evaluate the myocardium of patients with recent previous myocardial infarction (at least 3 months of age). Infarct size in the left ventricle of obese patients was found to be smaller than in those with normal body weight (11% ± 4% vs 16% ± 9%) with a P value of less than .03.

Finally, in a recent study by Lavie and colleagues,[20] a cohort of 529 patients in a cardiac rehabilitation program was evaluated. Survival analysis demonstrated that patients with a BMI of more than 35 had the lowest mortality risk. This study further demonstrated that this relationship persisted with respect to body composition, whereby patients with the highest baseline percent body fat had a lower mortality risk when compared with patients with a normal baseline body fat (2.8% vs 10.6%, respectively). Fonarow and colleagues[60] demonstrated a linear reduction in in-hospital mortality as the BMI increased. His findings showed a 10% reduction in mortality for every 5-unit increase in BMI.

SUMMARY

It is clear that obesity confers an overall decrease in lifetime survival. Many observations suggest that overweight patients survive better and live longer after cardiovascular stress and surgery than underweight or normal-weight individuals.

Current literature suggests a survival benefit for the obese that seems to be independent of age or sex difference, medical care, medical therapy, or other epidemiologic or environmental factors. Evidence suggests that some independent component of protection seems to be conferred by obesity alone.

The physiologic basic for this perceived benefit is currently conjecture. Nonetheless, some evidence suggests that metabolic activity and cellular physiologic changes in the obese might be adaptive for acute cardiovascular stress and in some chronic conditions.

Further study is required with wider populations, better markers, and improved prognostic factors for this to be fully elucidated. In the interim, the weight of evidence does not appear to be strong enough for us to advocate a more obese population.

REFERENCES

1. Curtis J, Selter J, Wang Y, et al. The obesity paradox. Arch Intern Med 2005;165: 55–61.
2. Lavie C, Milani R, Ventura H. Obesity and cardiovascular disease. J Am Coll Cardiol 2008;53:1925–32.
3. Hastie C, Padmanabhan S, Slack R, et al. Obesity paradox in a cohort of 4880 conceptive patient undergoing percutaneous coronary intervention. Eur Heart J 2010;31(2):222–6.
4. Romero-Corral A, Montori V, Somers V, et al. Association of bodyweight with total mortality and with cardiovascular events in coronary artery disease; a systematic review of cohort studies. Lancet 2006;368:666–78.
5. Adam H, Trichopoulos D. Obesity and mortality from cancer. N Engl J Med 2003; 348(17):1623–4.
6. Price G, Vavy R, Breeze E, et al. Weight, shape and mortality risk in older persons; elevated waist-hip ratio; height body mass index, is associated with a greater risk of death. Am J Clin 2006;84:449–60.
7. Flegal KM, Carroll MD, Ogden CL, et al. Prevalence and trends in obesity among US adults, 1999–2000. JAMA 2002;288(14):1723–7.
8. Yusuf S, Hanken S, Ounpuu S, et al. Obesity and the risk of myocardial infarction in 27,000 participants from 52 countries. A case-control study. Lancet 2005;366: 1640–9.
9. Faroogi S, Keogh J, Giles S, et al. Clinical spectrum of obesity and mutations in the melanocortin 4 receptor give. N Engl J Med 2003;348(12):1085–95.
10. Calle E, Rodriguez C, Walke-Thurmoid K, et al. Overweight obesity and mortality from cancer is a prospectively studied cohort of U.S. adults. N Engl J Med 2003; 348(17):625–38.
11. Roberts DL, Dive C, Renehan AG, et al. Biological mechanisms linking obesity and cancer risk: new perspectives. Annu Rev Med 2010;61:301–16.
12. Hall JE. The kidney, hypertension, and obesity. Hypertension 2003;41(3 Pt 2): 625–33.
13. Abir F, Bell R. Assessment and management of the obese patient. Crit Care Med 2004;32(Suppl):887–91.
14. Juan CC, Chuang TY, Lien CC, et al. Leptin increases endothelin type A receptor levels in vascular smooth muscle cells. Am J Physiol Endocrinol Metab 2008; 294(3):E481–7.
15. Cardillo C, Nambi SS, Kilcoyne CM, et al. Insulin stimulates both endothelin and nitric oxide activity in the human forearm. Circulation 1999;100:820–5.
16. Stamler R, Ford CE, Stamler J. Why do lean hypertensives have higher mortality rates than other hypertensives? Findings of the hypertension detection and follow-up program. Hypertension 1991;17(4):553–64.
17. Tuomilehto J. Body mass index and prognosis in elderly hypertensive patients: a report from the European Working Party on High Blood Pressure in the Elderly. Am J Med 1991;90(3A):34S–41S.

18. Wassertheil-Smoller S, Fann C, Allman RM, et al. Relation of low body mass to death and stroke in the systolic hypertension in the elderly program. The SHEP Cooperative Research Group. Arch Intern Med 2000;160(4):494–500.
19. Uretsky S, Messerli FH, Bangalore S, et al. Obesity paradox in patients with hypertension and coronary artery disease. Am J Med 2007;120(10):863–70.
20. Lavie C, Ventura H, Milani R. The obesity paradox: is smoking/lung disease the explanation. Chest 2008;134:896–8.
21. Lavie CJ, Milani RV, Artham SM, et al. The obesity paradox, weight loss, and coronary disease. Am J Med 2009;122(12):1106–14.
22. de Jong PE, Verhave JC, Pinto-Sietsma SJ, et al. PREVEND study group. Obesity and target organ damage: the kidney. Int J Obes Relat Metab Disord 2002; 26(Suppl 4):S21–4.
23. Foster MC, Hwang SJ, Larson MG, et al. Overweight, obesity, and the development of stage 3 CKD: the Framingham Heart Study. Am J Kidney Dis 2008; 52(1):39–48.
24. Degoulet P, Legrain M, Reach I, et al. Mortality risk factors in patients treated by chronic hemodialysis. Report of the Diaphane collaborative study. Nephron 1982; 31:103–10.
25. Leavey SF, McCullough K, Hecking E, et al. Body mass index and mortality in 'healthier' as compared with 'sicker' haemodialysis patients: results from the Dialysis Outcomes and Practice Patterns Study (DOPPS). Nephrol Dial Transplant 2001;16:2386–94.
26. Leavey SF, Strawderman RL, Jones CA, et al. Simple nutritional indicators as independent predictors of mortality in hemodialysis patients. Am J Kidney Dis 1998;31:997–1006.
27. Fleischmann E, Teal N, Dudley J, et al. Influence of excess weight on mortality and hospital stay in 1346 hemodialysis patients. Kidney Int 1999;55:1560–7.
28. Wong JS, Port FK, Hulbert-Shearon TE, et al. Survival advantage in Asian American end-stage renal disease patients. Kidney Int 1999;55:2515–23.
29. Abbott KC, Glanton CW, Trespalacios FC, et al. Body mass index, dialysis modality, and survival: analysis of the United States Renal Data System Dialysis Morbidity and Mortality Wave II Study. Kidney Int 2004;65:597–605.
30. Glanton CW, Hypolite IO, Hshieh PB, et al. Factors associated with improved short term survival in obese end stage renal disease patients. Ann Epidemiol 2003;13:136–43.
31. Kaizu Y, Tsunega Y, Yoneyama T, et al. Overweight as another nutritional risk factor for the long-term survival of non-diabetic hemodialysis patients. Clin Nephrol 1998;50:44–50.
32. Kutner NG, Zhang R. Body mass index as a predictor of continued survival in older chronic dialysis patients. Int Urol Nephrol 2001;32:441–8.
33. Canada-USA Peritoneal Dialysis Study Group. Adequacy of dialysis and nutrition in continuous peritoneal dialysis: association with clinical outcomes. J Am Soc Nephrol 1996;7:198–207.
34. Hakim RM, Lowrie E. Obesity and mortality in ESRD: is it good to be fat? Kidney Int 1999;55:1580–1.
35. Madero M, Sarnak M, Wang X, et al. Body mass index and mortality in CKD. Am J Kidney Dis 2007;50:1104–11.
36. McCusker FX, Teehan BP, Thorpe KE, et al. How much peritoneal dialysis is necessary for maintaining a good nutritional status? Kidney Int 1996;56(Suppl):S56–61.
37. Johnson DW, Herzig KA, Purdie DM, et al. Is obesity a favorable prognostic factor in peritoneal dialysis patients? Perit Dial Int 2000;20:715–21.

38. Chung SH, Lindholm B, Lee HB. Influence of initial nutritional status on continuous ambulatory peritoneal dialysis patient survival. Perit Dial Int 2000;20:19–26.

39. Snyder JJ, Foley RN, Gilbertson DT, et al. Body size and outcomes on peritoneal dialysis in the United States. Kidney Int 2003;64:1838–44.

40. McDonald SP, Collins JF, Johnson DW. Obesity is associated with worse peritoneal dialysis outcomes in the Australia and New Zealand patient populations. J Am Soc Nephrol 2003;14:2894–901.

41. Aslam N, Bernardini J, Fried L, et al. Large body mass index does not predict short-term survival in peritoneal dialysis patients. Perit Dial Int 2002;22:191–6.

42. Kalantar-Zadeh K, Abbott KC, Salahudeen AK, et al. Survival advantages of obesity in dialysis patients. Am J Clin Nutr 2005;81(3):543–54.

43. Vachharajani V. Influence of obesity on sepsis. Pathophysiology 2008;15(2): 123–34.

44. Borstein S, Licinic J, Tauchroitz R, et al. Plasma leptin levels are increased in survivors of acute sepsis. Associated loss of diurnal rhythm in cortisol and leptin secretion. J Clin Endocrinal Metab 1998;83:280–3.

45. Tsochitiasi H, Yamamoto K, Msoda K, et al. Circulating concentration of adiponectin on endogenous lipopolysaccharide neutralizing protein, decrease in rate with polymicrobial sepsis. J Surg Res 2006;134:348–53.

46. Sunden-Collberg, Nystrom T, Lee M, et al. Elevation of resistin correlates with severity of disease in severe sepsis and septic shock. Crit Care Med 2007;35: 1536–42.

47. El-Soth A, Sikka P, Borkanat K, et al. Morbid obesity in the medical ICU. Chest 2001;120:1989–97.

48. Nasraway S, Albert M, Donnelly A, et al. Morbid obesity is an independent determinant of death among surgical critically ill patients. Crit Care Med 2006;34: 964–70.

49. Newell M, Bard M, Gottler C, et al. Body mass index and outcomes in critically-ill injured blunt trauma patients: weighing the impact. J Am Coll Surg 2007;204: 1056–61.

50. Bercault N, Boulain T, Kateifan K, et al. Obesity-related excess mortality rate in an adult intensive care unit; a risk adjusted matched cohort study. Crit Care Med 2004;32:998–1008.

51. Yacqashi M, Jean R, Zuriquit M, et al. Outcome of morbid obesity in the intensive care unit. J Intensive Care Med 2005;20:147–54.

52. Akinnusi M, Pined L, El Soth A. Effect of obesity on intensive care morbidity and mortality a meta analysis. Crit Care Med 2008;36:151–8.

53. Mullen S, Moorman D, Davenport D. The obesity paradox, body mass index and outcome in patients undergoing non bariatric general surgery. Ann Surg 2009; 250(1):762–72.

54. Davenport D, Xenos E, Hosokawa P, et al. The influence of body mass index obesity status on vascular surgery 30-day morbidity and mortality. J Vasc Surg 2009;49:140–7.

55. Oreopaolus A, Padual R, Norris C, et al. Effect of obesity on short and long term mortality post-coronary revascularization; a meta-analysis. Obesity (Silver Spring) 2008;16:442–80.

56. Calle EE, Thun MJ, Petrelli JM, et al. Body-mass index and mortality in a prospective cohort of US adults. N Engl J Med 1999;341:1097–105.

57. Yusuf S, Hawken S, Ounpuu S, et al. Effect of potentially modifiable risk factors associated with myocardial infarction in 52 countries (the INTERHEART study): case-control study. Lancet 2004;364:937–52.

58. Arena R, Lavie CJ. The obesity paradox and outcome in hart failure: is excess body weight truly protective? Future Cardiol 2010;6(1):1–6.

59. Oreopoulos A, Padwal R, Kalantar-Zadeh K, et al. Body mass index and mortality in heart failure: a meta-analysis. Am Heart J 2008;156(1):13–22.

60. Fonarow GC, Srikanthan P, Costanzo MR, et al. An obesity paradox in acute heart failure: analysis of body mass index and in hospital mortality for 108927 patients in the Acute Decompensated Heart Failure National Registry. Am Heart J 2008; 153(1):74–81.

61. Horwich TB, Fonarow GC, Hamilton MA, et al. The relationship between obesity and mortality in patients with heart failure. J Am Coll Cardiol 2001;38:789–95.

62. Curtis JP, Selter JG, Wang Y, et al. The obesity paradox: body mass index and outcomes in patients with heart failure. Arch Intern Med 2005;165:55–61.

63. Mehta RH, Califf RM, Garg J, et al. The impact of anthropomorphic outcomes in patients with myocardial infarction. Eur Heart J 2007;28:415–24.

64. Gurm HS, Brennan DM, Booth J, et al. Impact of body mass index on outcome after percutaneous coronary intervention (the obesity paradox). Am J Cardiol 2002;90:42–5.

65. Gruberg L, Weissman NJ, Waksman R, et al. The impact of obesity on the short-term and long-term outcomes after percutaneous coronary intervention: the obesity paradox? J Am Coll Cardiol 2002;39:578–84.

Pulmonary System and Obesity

Doyle D. Ashburn, DO[a], Angela DeAntonio, MD, FCCP[b],
Mary Jane Reed, MD, FCCM, FCCP[a],*

KEYWORDS

- Pulmonary • Obesity • Respiratory failure • Lung mechanics
- Mechanical ventilation • ARDS

There are several challenges in the management of respiratory failure in the obese population. Pulmonary physiology is significantly altered leading to reduced lung volumes, decreased compliance, abnormal ventilation and perfusion relationships, and respiratory muscle inefficiency.[1] These complications lead to a prolonged requirement for mechanical ventilation and increased intensive-care-unit (ICU) length of stay.[2,3]

LUNG VOLUMES

Lung volumes are appreciably affected by obesity. Most reported is a decrease in functional residual capacity (FRC) and expiratory reserve volume (ERV).[4,5] An inverse relationship between body mass index (BMI) and FRC has been established[4,5] with modest increases in BMI leading to decreased FRC and ERV.[4] Vital capacity (VC), total lung capacity (TLC), and residual volume (RV) can also be reduced but to a lesser extent. Jones and Nzekwu[4] studied the effect of obesity on lung volumes in association with BMI and noted a 0.5% decrease in VC, TLC, and RV for each unit increase in BMI as compared with a 3% and 5% decrease in FRC and ERV, respectively. The increase in adipose tissue around the rib cage and abdomen leads to decreased chest wall compliance and increased resistance, which in turn increases the mass load on the respiratory musculature and significantly reduces FRC.[6] These changes are even more notable in the supine position because of the impedance of the diaphragm by the abdomen.[7] As the FRC decreases it approaches the closing capacity, which can lead to airway closure within the range of tidal breathing. Areas of lung may be underventilated leading to intrapulmonary shunting and hypoxemia.[8,9]

Disclosure statement: The authors have nothing to disclose.
[a] Department of Critical Care Medicine, Geisinger Medical Center, 100 North Academy Avenue, Danville, PA 17822, USA
[b] Department of Critical Care Medicine, Geisinger Wyoming Valley Medical Center, 1000 East Mountain Drive, Wilkes-Barre, PA 18711, USA
* Corresponding author.
E-mail address: mreed@geisinger.edu

Crit Care Clin 26 (2010) 597–602
doi:10.1016/j.ccc.2010.06.008
0749-0704/10/$ – see front matter © 2010 Published by Elsevier Inc.

criticalcare.theclinics.com

LUNG MECHANICS

Another important alteration in respiratory physiology of patients who are obese is an overall stiffening of the respiratory system. Pulmonary compliance is significantly reduced in these patients and can be reduced up to 42% in patients with obesity hypoventilation syndrome.[10] This loss of compliance has been demonstrated in multiple studies and appears to be exponentially related to BMI.[5] There are several mechanisms contributing to the decrease in lung and chest wall compliance.[1] Reduced lung compliance is in part caused by an increase in the volume of blood within the pulmonary circulation,[11] but mostly is a function of decreased volumes. The lower the FRC the more it approaches the closing capacity of the smaller airways causing collapse and atelectasis.[9] These lower volumes also increase alveolar surface tension leading to decreased compliance.[12]

Several authors report that increased adipose tissue around the ribs, diaphragm, and abdomen leads to a decrease in chest wall compliance[1,5,6] and has been reported to be more pronounced in the supine position.[6] It has also been postulated that the reduction in compliance is caused by lower volumes and that obese subjects are breathing over a less compliant area of the thoracic volume-pressure curve.[10] The data regarding chest wall compliance remains variable because several studies have shown little or no effect on overall pulmonary compliance, stressing more of a reduction in lung compliance as the major factor.[5,13,14] Despite the controversy in the literature, which may be secondary to differences in technique, it seems logical that increased mass loading on the chest affects respiratory mechanics negatively, possibly because of irreversible closure or collapse of alveolar units leading to decreased lung compliance.[10]

Further compounding the increased work of breathing in obese individuals is increased airway resistance. The cross-sectional area of the upper airway is reduced because of increased parapharyngeal fat deposition. These airways are also more prone to collapse, especially at lower lung volumes as is seen with increased BMI.[15,16] The smaller airways are also affected. Rubinstein and colleagues[17] found higher levels of pulmonary resistance, a decrease in forced expiratory volume in the first second of expiration (FEV_1), and decreased flow rates in obese versus nonobese individuals. This finding suggested that change in airway caliber may be representative of remodeling from inflammatory adipocytokines or damage from repeated opening and closing of the airways during tidal respirations.[18]

VENTILATION AND PERFUSION

Obesity has been associated with changes in ventilation and perfusion (V/Q) matching. In normal pulmonary physiology the distribution of regional ventilation and perfusion is predominantly in the lower, dependant lung zones. In obesity the lower lung zones are also predominantly perfused, but ventilation is preferentially distributed to the upper lung zones.[19,20] It is thought that these changes are likely caused by small airway closure caused by lower ERV[19] and possibly related to extrinsic factors affecting chest wall and diaphragm function,[20] which can lead to V/Q mismatching and hypoxemia. These changes are more pronounced in the supine and lateral decubitus positions, and an inverse relationship between BMI and the partial pressure of oxygen in the inferior pulmonary vein while in the supine position has been identified.[21]

RESPIRATORY MUSCLE INEFFICIENCY

Obesity leads to decreased endurance of the muscles of respiration and increased oxygen consumption (VO2) by those muscles. It is estimated that the maximum voluntary ventilation (MVV) is reduced by 20% in healthy obese individuals and up to 45% in people with obesity hypoventilation syndrome.[1,6,22] Increased load on the respiratory system by adipose tissue is the likely cause for this finding. Kress and colleagues[23] studied VO2 in obese subjects before and during general anesthesia, which focused mainly on the respiratory component (VO2resp), and noted a 5-fold increase in VO2 with obesity. It has been estimated that there is up to a 10-fold greater increase in VO2 with obesity hypoventilation syndrome.[6] One can see how this lack of respiratory reserve would put the morbidly obese at an increased risk for respiratory failure when under the stress associated with critical illness.

RESPIRATORY FAILURE AND MECHANICAL VENTILATION

Acute lung injury (ALI) is defined as acute onset of bilateral pulmonary infiltrates, a partial pressure of oxygen (pO2) to fraction of inspired oxygen (FiO2) ratio less than 300, and a lack of pulmonary venous hypertension (ie, pulmonary capillary wedge pressure less than 18 mmHg). Acute respiratory distress syndrome (ARDS) is ALI with a pO2 to FiO2 ratio less than 200.[24] ALI/ARDS are commonly seen in critical illness and carry a significant mortality.[25] The physiologic alterations seen in the respiratory systems of obese patients pose significant challenges for management.

ALI/ARDS causes a decrease in lung compliance because of the inflammatory changes in the lung parenchyma, hyaline formation in the alveoli, a decrease in surfactant activity, and regional alveolar collapse.[25] Lung compliance is already reduced in the obese population as previously outlined. These changes in compliance lead to abnormally high airway pressures during mechanical ventilation. High transpulmonary pressures (the difference in pressure between the alveoli and the pleural space, which is the distending pressure of the lung) in ALI/ARDS lead to over distension of the alveoli and further lung injury termed *ventilator-induced lung injury*.[26] Typically the goal is to keep plateau pressures (an estimate of alveolar pressure) less than 30 cm of water; this may be difficult in the obese individual. One aspect of this to keep in mind is the contribution of the chest wall compliance to the total respiratory compliance. As discussed, increased adipose tissue around the ribs, diaphragm, and abdomen leads to a decrease in compliance and increased pleural pressure thus decreasing the transpulmonary pressure in the obese. This decrease may be lung protective, allowing higher plateau pressures to be tolerated in these patients.[27] Several studies have shown that using a low-volume strategy for ventilation in ALI/ARDS in an attempt to decrease airway pressures and over distension of the lung reduces mortality, most notably a large trial by the Acute Respiratory Distress Syndrome Network.[25,28] From the results of this trial a recommendation for tidal volume is to use 6 mL/Kg, or lower based on plateau pressures. It is especially important to use ideal body weight when calculating a goal tidal volume with obese patients because the size of the lung does not change appreciably with weight gain.[7]

It has been proposed that repeated opening and closing of small airways during tidal respirations is another mechanism of ventilator-induced lung injury, termed *atelectrauma*.[26] As previously outlined obese individuals have a lower FRC approaching the closing capacity of the small airways leading to their collapse. They tend to have significant atelectasis, especially in the supine position. Positive end expiratory pressure (PEEP) can be applied to counteract this and help maintain FRC. The benefit of PEEP in mechanical ventilation has been realized since the 1970s.[29] In recent years there has been great interest in what the optimum PEEP is, especially in obesity. Pelosi and colleagues[30] demonstrated improved oxygenation with PEEP at 10 cm of water in obese subjects versus nonobese subjects when undergoing abdominal surgery.

Several more recent studies have also shown benefit at this level.[31–33] Erlandsson and colleagues[34] studied impedance tomography with varying levels of PEEP in subjects with BMI greater than 40 and found a level of 15 cm of water to be optimal. The majority of studies have been done in surgical subjects looking at intraoperative atelectasis and lung volumes; there is a paucity of data regarding PEEP and obesity outside of the anesthesia literature. Despite this, it seems logical that given the lower FRC, collapse of dependant lung, and decreased chest wall compliance higher levels of PEEP would be beneficial in the obese population. One could argue that this may cause worsening hemodynamic instability. Erlandsson and colleagues[34] used volume expansion to counteract this and it has been theorized that opening of atelectatic lung segments may actually decrease pulmonary vascular resistance and improve cardiac output.[35] Also, a recent study looking at higher levels of PEEP, termed *open-lung ventilation* versus lower levels showed no difference in adverse affects or mortality between the groups, although morbidly obese individuals were excluded from this study.[36]

The position of obese patients also plays a significant role in ventilatory management. Yamane and colleagues[21] noted hypoxemia in the inferior pulmonary veins in obese subjects when supine. This finding is thought to be related to collapse of regional lung segments in the dependent areas of the lung. Increased impedance of the diaphragm leading to decreased lung volumes in the supine position contributes to the atelectasis. Burns and colleagues[37] studied body position and tidal volumes and respiratory rate in obese individuals. They noted higher tidal volumes and lower spontaneous respiratory rates when subjects were placed in a 45° reverse Trendelenburg position as compared with 90° upright posture. Boyce and colleagues[38] looked at the ideal body positioning in the perioperative period and noted a longer period to desaturation with subjects in a 30° reverse Trendelenburg when compared with supine or 30° upright position. This finding would suggest that the ideal positioning for obese patients on mechanical ventilation is reverse Trendelenburg when there are no contraindications present.

It would seem reasonable to think that obesity would increase mortality in the ICU but in fact the data supports the contrary.[2,39–41] O'Brien and colleagues[40] noted that BMI was an independent predictor of mortality in the ICU, but it was the subjects that had a low BMI that were at the most risk. What these studies did show was obesity is related to a prolonged duration of mechanical ventilation and ICU length of stay. Morris and colleagues[41] studied this population and found an increase in morbidity identified as more days on the vent and longer ICU stays. They also reported that these subjects were more likely to be discharged to rehabilitation facilities or skilled nursing facilities suggesting morbidity that extends beyond the hospital.[35]

REFERENCES

1. Parameswaran K, Todd DC, Soth M. Altered respiratory physiology in obesity. Can Respir J 2006;13(4):203–10.
2. Akinnusi ME, Pineda LA, El Solh AA. Effect of obesity on intensive care morbidity and mortality: a meta-analysis. Crit Care Med 2008;36(1):151–8.
3. Oliveros H, Villamor E. Obesity and mortality in critically ill adults: a systematic review and meta-analysis. Obesity (Silver Spring) 2008;16(3):515–21.
4. Jones RL, Nzekwu MM. The effects of body mass index on lung volumes. Chest 2006;130(3):827–33.
5. Pelosi P, Croci M, Ravagnan I, et al. The effects of body mass on lung volumes, respiratory mechanics, and gas exchange during general anesthesia. Anesth Analg 1998;87(3):654–60.

6. Koenig SM. Pulmonary complications of obesity. Am J Med Sci 2001;321(4): 249–79.
7. Malhotra A, Hillman D. Obesity and the lung: 3. Obesity, respiration and intensive care. Thorax 2008;63(10):925–31.
8. Benedik PS, Baun MM, Keus L, et al. Effects of body position on resting lung volume in overweight and mildly to moderately obese subjects. Respir Care 2009;54(3):334–9.
9. Hedenstierna G, McCarthy G, Bergstrom M. Airway closure during mechanical ventilation. Anesthesiology 1976;44(2):114–23.
10. Sharp JT, Henry JP, Sweany SK, et al. The total work of breathing in normal and obese men. J Clin Invest 1964;43:728–39.
11. Naimark A, Cherniack RM. Compliance of the respiratory system and its components in health and obesity. J Appl Physiol 1960;15:377–82.
12. Behazin N, Jones SB, Cohen RI, et al. Respiratory restriction and elevated pleural and esophageal pressures in morbid obesity. J Appl Physiol 2010;108(1):212–8.
13. Hedenstierna G, Santesson J. Breathing mechanics, dead space and gas exchange in the extremely obese, breathing spontaneously and during anaesthesia with intermittent positive pressure ventilation. Acta Anaesthesiol Scand 1976;20(3):248–54.
14. Suratt PM, Wilhoit SC, Hsiao HS, et al. Compliance of chest wall in obese subjects. J Appl Physiol 1984;57(2):403–7.
15. Shelton KE, Woodson H, Gay S, et al. Pharyngeal fat in obstructive sleep apnea. Am Rev Respir Dis 1993;148(2):462–6.
16. Bradley TD, Brown IG, Grossman RF, et al. Pharyngeal size in snorers, nonsnorers, and patients with obstructive sleep apnea. N Engl J Med 1986;315(21): 1327–31.
17. Rubinstein I, Zamel N, DuBarry L, et al. Airflow limitation in morbidly obese, nonsmoking men. Ann Intern Med 1990;112(11):828–32.
18. Salome CM, King GG, Berend N. Physiology of obesity and effects on lung function. J Appl Physiol 2010;108(1):206–11.
19. Holley HS, Milic-Emili J, Becklake MR, et al. Regional distribution of pulmonary ventilation and perfusion in obesity. J Clin Invest 1967;46(4):475–81.
20. Demedts M. Regional distribution of lung volumes and of gas inspired at residual volume: influence of age, body weight and posture. Bull Eur Physiopathol Respir 1980;16(3):271–85.
21. Yamane T, Date T, Tokuda M, et al. Hypoxemia in inferior pulmonary veins in supine position is dependent on obesity. Am J Respir Crit Care Med 2008; 178(3):295–9.
22. Ray CS, Sue DY, Bray G, et al. Effects of obesity on respiratory function. Am Rev Respir Dis 1983;128(3):501–6.
23. Kress JP, Pohlman AS, Alverdy J, et al. The impact of morbid obesity on oxygen cost of breathing (VO(2RESP)) at rest. Am J Respir Crit Care Med 1999;160(3): 883–6.
24. Bernard GR, Artigas A, Brigham KL, et al. Report of the American-European Consensus conference on acute respiratory distress syndrome: definitions, mechanisms, relevant outcomes, and clinical trial coordination. Consensus Committee. J Crit Care 1994;9(1):72–81.
25. Malhotra A. Low-tidal-volume ventilation in the acute respiratory distress syndrome. N Engl J Med 2007;357(11):1113–20.
26. Dreyfuss D, Saumon G. Ventilator-induced lung injury: lessons from experimental studies. Am J Respir Crit Care Med 1998;157(1):294–323.

27. Hess DR, Bigatello LM. The chest wall in acute lung injury/acute respiratory distress syndrome. Curr Opin Crit Care 2008;14(1):94–102.
28. The Acute Respiratory Distress Syndrome Network. Ventilation with lower tidal volumes as compared with traditional tidal volumes for acute lung injury and the acute respiratory distress syndrome. N Engl J Med 2000;342:1301–8.
29. Webb HH, Tierney DF. Experimental pulmonary edema due to intermittent positive pressure ventilation with high inflation pressures. Protection by positive end-expiratory pressure. Am Rev Respir Dis 1974;110(5):556–65.
30. Pelosi P, Ravagnan I, Giurati G, et al. Positive end-expiratory pressure improves respiratory function in obese but not in normal subjects during anesthesia and paralysis. Anesthesiology 1999;91(5):1221–31.
31. Reinius H, Jonsson L, Gustafsson S, et al. Prevention of atelectasis in morbidly obese patients during general anesthesia and paralysis: a computerized tomography study. Anesthesiology 2009;111(5):979–87.
32. Talab HF, Zabani IA, Abdelrahman HS, et al. Intraoperative ventilatory strategies for prevention of pulmonary atelectasis in obese patients undergoing laparoscopic bariatric surgery. Anesth Analg 2009;109(5):1511–6.
33. Valenza F, Vagginelli F, Tiby A, et al. Effects of the beach chair position, positive end-expiratory pressure, and pneumoperitoneum on respiratory function in morbidly obese patients during anesthesia and paralysis. Anesthesiology 2007; 107(5):725–32.
34. Erlandsson K, Odenstedt H, Lundin S, et al. Positive end-expiratory pressure optimization using electric impedance tomography in morbidly obese patients during laparoscopic gastric bypass surgery. Acta Anaesthesiol Scand 2006; 50(7):833–9.
35. Gernoth C, Wagner G, Pelosi P, et al. Respiratory and haemodynamic changes during decremental open lung positive end-expiratory pressure titration in patients with acute respiratory distress syndrome. Crit Care 2009;13(2):R59.
36. Meade MO, Cook DJ, Guyatt GH, et al. Ventilation strategy using low tidal volumes, recruitment maneuvers, and high positive end-expiratory pressure for acute lung injury and acute respiratory distress syndrome: a randomized controlled trial. JAMA 2008;299(6):637–45.
37. Burns SM, Egloff MB, Ryan B, et al. Effect of body position on spontaneous respiratory rate and tidal volume in patients with obesity, abdominal distension and ascites. Am J Crit Care 1994;3(2):102–6.
38. Boyce JR, Ness T, Castroman P, et al. A preliminary study of the optimal anesthesia positioning for the morbidly obese patient. Obes Surg 2003;13(1):4–9.
39. Hogue CW Jr, Stearns JD, Colantuoni E, et al. The impact of obesity on outcomes after critical illness: a meta-analysis. Intensive Care Med 2009;35(7):1152–70.
40. O'Brien JM Jr, Phillips GS, Ali NA, et al. Body mass index is independently associated with hospital mortality in mechanically ventilated adults with acute lung injury. Crit Care Med 2006;34(3):738–44.
41. Morris AE, Stapleton RD, Rubenfeld GD, et al. The association between body mass index and clinical outcomes in acute lung injury. Chest 2007;131(2):342–8.

Cardiovascular Considerations in Critically Ill Obese Patients

Mitchell K. Craft, DO[a], Mary Jane Reed, MD, FCCM, FCCP[b],*

KEYWORDS

- Obesity • Critical illness • Obesity cardiomyopathy
- Heart failure

The spectrum of cardiovascular alterations in obese patients is rather intricate, making management during their critical illness complex. As the obesity epidemic evolves, it is prudent to identify and consider these changes during management of these patients. As will be discussed, these changes affect: circulatory volumes, cardiac structure and dysfunction, electrocardiographic findings, and changes at the cellular level.

The relationship between obesity and stroke volume has been well elucidated. As weight increases beyond ideal body weight, there is a linear increase in total blood volume. With this is a direct increase in cardiac output, almost exclusively dependent on increased stroke volume, with resting heart rates remaining unchanged. In resting, normotensive obese patients, systemic vascular resistance has been noted to be normal or reduced.[1–6] It is suggested that the increase in cardiac output is consequence of increasing metabolic requirements of excessive adiposity. As derived by left and right heart catheterization data, De Divitiis and colleagues[4] described an increased oxygen consumption that directly correlated with increased weight, yet maintaining a normal A-maximum oxygen consumption (VO_2). In addition, obesity is associated with an increased fat-free mass, which also has been correlated to an increased stroke volume and cardiac output.

Obesity has been associated with various electrocardiographic and echocardiograph findings. Several series have shown disproportionate frequency of: leftward shifts of P wave, QRS and T wave axes, left ventricular (LV) hypertrophy patterns, low voltage, prolonged QT interval, and ST-T abnormalities. It appears that many of

[a] Department of Critical Care Medicine, Geisinger Medical Center, 100 North Academy Avenue, Danville, PA 17822, USA
[b] Departments of General Surgery and Critical Care Medicine, Geisinger Medical Center, Temple University Medical School, 100 North Academy Avenue, Mail Code: 20-37, Danville, PA 17822, USA
* Corresponding author.
E-mail address: mreed@geisinger.edu

Crit Care Clin 26 (2010) 603–605
doi:10.1016/j.ccc.2010.06.003   criticalcare.theclinics.com
0749-0704/10/$ – see front matter © 2010 Published by Elsevier Inc.

the alterations can normalize with weight loss.[7–9] Echocardiography is often challenging in the obese patient due to limitations in adequacy of images. As noted previously, there is an increased blood volume, which translates to a persistently increased preload and increased wall tension. As a result, there is LV hypertrophy and dilation. In normotensive patients, this is primarily eccentric hypertrophy. Obese patients, however, are at increased risk for systemic hypertension, and concentric hypertrophy remains common. With increasing LV mass, there is decreased compliance; several echocardiography studies implicate obesity as an independent risk factor for left atrial enlargement and LV diastolic dysfunction.[5,10–13] In addition, LV systolic dysfunction (obesity cardiomyopathy) may be identified when the LV dilation exceeds the compensatory effects of the left ventricular hypertrophy.[10] The increased cardiac output also may result in right ventricular (RV) hypertrophy/enlargement. Pulmonary arterial hypertension may be present as an isolated finding or coupled with the previously stated RV abnormalities. This is often a result of obesity-related diseases, obstructive sleep apnea, and obesity hypoventilation syndrome.

Obesity has been associated with an increased risk of heart failure, with additional risks associated with critical illness. As illustrated by the Framingham Group, after excluding the effects of conventional risk factors, obesity was associated with a 5% to 7% increased risk of heart failure per 1% increase in body-mass index.[14] As there are many analogous physiologic responses to critical illness as to exercise, it may be reasonable to extrapolate the cardiac effects seen with exercise to critically ill obese patients. With stress both LV systolic and diastolic dysfunctions have been noted. Furthermore, exercise results in increased LV end diastolic pressures and pulmonary capillary wedge pressures.[4,15,16] In dealing with critically ill patients, large volume shifts and aggressive fluid resuscitation are commonplace, and a propensity for acute pulmonary edema ought to be recognized. Further complications may arise from the disproportionate prevalence of atrial fibrillation in obese patients, which will further impair cardiac function.[17] On a cellular level, associations with cardiac dysfunction have been made with: decreased lymphocyte beta-adrenergic receptors, cardiodepressant factors released from adipocytes, and alterations in neuroendocrine pathways.[18,19]

With a growing obese population, preventative and therapeutic strategies need to be developed to combat the complex cardiac pathophysiology related to obesity. This is paramount in the management of critically ill obese patients.

REFERENCES

1. Alexander J, Dennis E, Smith W, et al. Blood volume, cardiac output, and distribution of systemic blood flow in extreme obesity. Cardiovasc Res Cent Bull 1962–1963;1:39–44.
2. Messerli F. Cardiovascular effects of obesity and hypertension. Lancet 1982; 319(82):1165–8.
3. Vaughan R, Conahan T. Part I:cardiopulmonary consequences of morbid obesity. Life Sci 1980;26:2119–27.
4. De Divitiis O, Fazio S, Petitto M, et al. Obesity and cardiac function. Circulation 1981;64(3):477–82.
5. Backman L, Freyschuss U, Hallbert D, et al. Cardiovascular function in extreme obesity. Acta Med Scand 1983;149:437–9.
6. Collis T, Devereux R, Roman M, et al. Relations of stroke volume and cardiac output to body composition. The strong heart study. Circulation 2001;103:820–5.

7. Fraley M, Birchem J, Senkottaiyan N, et al. Obesity and the electrocardiogram. Obes Rev 2005;6(4):275–81.
8. Frank S, Colliver J, Frank A. The electrocardiogram in obesity: statistical analysis of 1029 patients. J Am Coll Cardiol 1986;7:295–9.
9. Alpert M, Terry B, Hamm C, et al. Effect of weight loss on the ECG of normotensive morbidly obese patients. Chest 2001;119:507–10.
10. Alport M. Obesity cardiomyopathy: pathophysiology and evolution of the clinical syndrome. Am J Med Sci 2001;321:225–36.
11. Rider O, Francis J, Ali M, et al. Determinants of left ventricular mass in obesity; a cardiovascular magnetic resonance study. J Cardiovasc Magn Reson 2009; 11(1):9.
12. Alport M, Lambert C, Taryy B, et al. Influence of left ventricular mass on diastolic filling in normotensive morbid obesity. Am Heart J 1995;130:1068–73.
13. Stritke J, Markus M, Duderstadt S, et al. The aging process of the heart: obesity is the main risk factor for left atrial enlargement during aging. J Am Coll Cardiol 2009;54(21):1982–9.
14. Kenchaiah S, Evans J, Levy D, et al. Obesity and the risk of heart failure. N Engl J Med 2002;347(5):305–13.
15. Alport M, Singh A, Terry B, et al. Effect of exercise on left ventricular systolic function and reserve in morbid obesity. Am J Cardiol 1989;63:1478.
16. Alpert M, Terry B, Mulekar M, et al. Cardiac morphology and left ventricular function in normotensive morbidly obese patients with and without congestive heart failure, and effect of weight loss. Am J Cardiol 1997;80:736–40.
17. Wang T, Parise H, Levy D, et al. Obesity and the risk of new-onset atrial fibrillation. JAMA 2004;292:2471–7.
18. Merlino G, Scaglione R, Paterna S, et al. Lymphocyte beta-adrenergic receptors in young subjects with peripheral or central obesity: relationship with central haemodynamics and left ventricular function. Eur Heart J 1994;15(6):786–92.
19. Lamounier-Zepter V, Look C, Alvarez J, et al. Adipocyte fatty acid-binding protein suppresses cardiomyocyte contraction. Circ Res 2009;105:326–34.

Acute Kidney Injury in the Critically Ill, Morbidly Obese Patient: Diagnostic and Therapeutic Challenges in a Unique Patient Population

Ion D. Bucaloiu, MD[a],*, Robert M. Perkins, MD[a,b],
William DiFilippo, MD[a], Taher Yahya, MD[a], Evan Norfolk, MD[a]

KEYWORDS

- Kidney • Injury • Morbid • Obesity • Critical
- Glomerular filtration rate

Acute kidney injury (AKI) is a common and serious complication in patients who are hospitalized, affecting up to 15.3% of all inpatients[1,2] and up to 25% of the critically ill population.[3] Despite the observation that the obese (body mass index [BMI], calculated as the weight in kilograms divided by the height in meters squared, >30) and morbidly obese (MO) (BMI >40) patients who are hospitalized represent growing fractions of the overall population in the intensive care unit (ICU) (as much as 30%[4,5] and 7%,[5] respectively), the incidence of AKI in the critically ill MO population is not known. This absence of information is surprising, given the well-recognized mortality risk conferred by an episode of AKI[6–11] and even more so when the typical burden of comorbid illness among MO patients is considered.

Why might the MO patient population warrant an analytical perspective distinct from the nonobese population? First, morbid obesity is an independent risk factor for

Funding support: None.

The authors state that they do not have any conflicts of interest.

[a] Department of Nephrology, Geisinger Medical Center, 100 North Academy Avenue, Danville, PA 17822, USA

[b] Biostatistics Research and Data Core, Henry Hood Center for Health Research, Danville, PA 17822, USA

* Corresponding author.

E-mail address: IDBUCALOIU@geisinger.edu

Crit Care Clin 26 (2010) 607–624

doi:10.1016/j.ccc.2010.06.005

0749-0704/10/$ – see front matter © 2010 Elsevier Inc. All rights reserved.

chronic kidney disease (CKD),[12–14] which in turn, in a nonobese population at least, is a risk factor for AKI.[15] Second, glomerular hyperfiltration expressed by a supranormal glomerular filtration rate (GFR)[16,17] is commonly seen in MO patients and may mask underlying chronic renal damage. Obesity-related glomerulopathy[18] is manifested as glomerulomegaly, mesangial expansion, and secondary focal and segmental glomerulosclerosis. This disease state may place the critically ill MO patients at higher risk for developing AKI because of preexisting glomerular pathologic conditions and lack of appropriate recognition by the provider of underlying renal damage resulting in inadequate prophylaxis (eg, for contrast-induced nephropathy) or inappropriate prescription of nephrotoxic medications (nonsteroidal anti-inflammatory agents, aminoglycosides, or others). Finally, the distinct histologic characteristics of chronic renal damage combined with the unique set of comorbid illnesses often present in critically ill MO patients, further raising the possibility of a unique set of risk factors for AKI in this population.

This article examines the available literature that reviews the limited epidemiologic analyses of AKI in the MO population, discusses the limitations of the available tools used in the estimation of GFR in this population, and describes patterns of injury that may be more prevalent in this cohort as compared with the nonobese population. Finally, the authors address the challenge of providing appropriate renal replacement therapy (RRT) to the MO patient in the ICU.

EPIDEMIOLOGY OF AKI IN MO CRITICALLY ILL PATIENTS

AKI complicates about 15% of all hospitalizations and is associated with excess mortality, increased length of stay, and increased health care costs.[19] In response to the limitations created by the myriad of definitions of AKI in the literature and because of the increased awareness that small increases in serum creatinine levels in patients who are hospitalized are associated with excess morbidity and mortality,[20] the Risk, Injury, Failure, Loss, End-stage renal disease (RIFLE) and Acute Kidney Injury Network (AKIN) criteria for the diagnosis of AKI have been recently created and validated.[10,21,22] In studies of critically ill patients, AKI is associated with mortality rates up to 50% to 60%.[3,11,23] By contrast, obesity in the critically ill may paradoxically confer a lower risk of in-hospital and long-term mortality.[4,24] The relationship between AKI, BMI, and mortality in critically ill patients has not been rigorously evaluated.

The incidence of AKI in a general hospitalized population varies depending on the diagnostic criteria used.[20,25] The application of the RIFLE criteria has yielded substantially larger incidence rates of AKI than previously cited in the literature.[20,26] In the general critically ill population, up to 67% of patients qualify as having AKI based on RIFLE criteria,[10] with one-third developing AKI within the first 48 hours of ICU admission.[27]

The incidence of AKI in the critically ill MO population is unknown despite 1 in 4 critically ill patients being MO.[28] The largest epidemiologic studies of AKI in the critically ill did not include subset analyses of this patient population.[3,11,23,29,30] Most available data on AKI in MO patients are limited and derived primarily from postoperative observational cohorts and with one exception[5] are not solely inclusive of patients who required intensive care admission. The incidence of postoperative AKI in MO patients varies between 2.8% and 14.3%, depending on the definition of AKI used, type of surgery performed, and the population studied (**Table 1**).[31–35] Nasraway and colleagues[5] evaluated the effect of morbid obesity on mortality in a prospective cohort of 1373 critically ill surgical patients. In addition to finding an independent relationship between a BMI greater than 40 and mortality, the investigators found that the

Table 1
Published studies reporting on the incidence of AKI in MO patients (BMI >40)

Investigators	Number of MO Patients	Definition of AKI Used	Study Design	Setting	Incidence of AKI (%)
McCullough et al,[31] 2006	109	An increase in baseline serum creatinine level >25% from baseline or an absolute increase of 0.5 mg/dL at any time during the hospital stay after surgery	Retrospective	Laparoscopic Roux-en-Y gastric bypass surgery	6 (5.5)
Sharma et al,[32] 2006	1800	An increase in serum creatinine level to >1.4 mg/dL or a relative increase of >0.3 mg/dL from baseline during the first postoperative week	Retrospective	Laparoscopic Roux-en-Y gastric bypass surgery	52 (2.8)
Thakar et al,[33] 2007	491	>50% increase in serum creatinine level relative to baseline during the first 3 postoperative days or requirement of dialysis during the postoperative period	Retrospective	Gastric bypass (open and laparoscopic)	42 (8.5)
Nasraway et al,[5] 2006	94	Serum creatinine >2 mg/dL	Prospective cohort	Surgical ICU	9 (9.6)
Wigfield et al,[34] 2006	1920	An increase in the levels of serum creatinine twice the baseline value and >2.0 mmol/L	Retrospective	Cardiac surgery (excluding cardiac transplantation and ventricular assist device surgeries)	11 (3)
Yap et al,[35] 2007	214	At least 2 of the following: raised serum creatinine level >200 μmol/L, doubling or greater increase in creatinine level compared with preoperative value, or new requirement for dialysis or hemofiltration	Retrospective	Cardiac surgery (coronary artery bypass and valvular surgery)	18 (8.4)

incidence of AKI (creatinine levels >2 mg/dL) in MO patients was 9.9% and was not significantly different from that of the nonobese group.

Risk factors for development of AKI after gastric bypass include age greater than 50 years, male gender, BMI greater than 50, preoperative CKD, diabetes, hypertension, presence of peripheral edema, operative time longer than 210 minutes,[32] and poor preoperative cardiopulmonary fitness.[31] In multivariate analysis, hyperlipidemia, preoperative use of angiotensin-converting enzyme inhibitor/angiotensin receptor blocker, and higher BMI were independently associated with increased incidence of AKI.[33] Consistent with reported studies in the nonobese population, patients who developed AKI had a higher hospital mortality (4.8% vs 0%, $P = .007$) and a longer length of hospitalization (4.0 vs 2.7 days, $P = .0003$) than controls.[33] Whether these findings can be confirmed in a critically ill (medical and/or surgical) MO population remains to be seen.

In a retrospective analysis of 1920 consecutive patients who underwent cardiac surgery, Wigfield and colleagues[34] observed a significantly increased incidence of AKI in MO patients compared with nonobese controls (14.3% vs 5.0%, $P = .003$). Despite the increase in the incidence of AKI, there was no significant difference in perioperative or 30-day mortality compared with the nonobese patients.[34] Yap and colleagues[35] performed a retrospective review of 11,736 patients who underwent cardiac surgery in Australia. Morbid obesity was present in 1.8% of this population and was associated with increased risks of postoperative ICU admission (adjusted odds ratio [OR] 2.2; 95% confidence interval [CI], 1.2–4.1), postoperative renal failure (adjusted OR 2.9; 95% CI, 1.7–4.9), and prolonged need for mechanical ventilation (adjusted OR 2.4; 95% CI, 1.6–3.7). The incidence of postoperative renal failure (defined as the presence of at least 2 of the following conditions: increased serum creatinine levels >200 μmol/L, doubling of serum creatinine levels compared with preoperative value, or initiation of RRT) was significantly higher in MO patients as compared with patients of normal weight (8.4% vs 4.4%, $P = .006$).

Despite the limitations of these studies, several important points regarding AKI in the MO are evident. First, postoperative AKI is not uncommon in this population. The incidence of AKI may be higher in critically ill obese individuals, especially when the more sensitive RIFLE/AKIN criteria are used to make the diagnosis as noted in the general population.[20] Second, in the postoperative period, MO patients are at increased risk of requiring intensive care admission. Third, identified risk factors for postoperative AKI in the MO population are similar to those observed in the general population. Finally, BMI itself is associated with postoperative AKI in MO patients. Whether these or other factors also predict AKI in any critically ill MO patient remains an open question. Given the growing recognition that the MO patients who are hospitalized represent a physiologically and clinically unique group, further epidemiologic research of this population is warranted.

GFR ESTIMATION IN CRITICALLY ILL OBESE PATIENTS, AND THE DIAGNOSIS OF AKI

Accurate assessment of GFR is essential for the diagnosis and treatment of AKI, for safe and effective drug dosing and monitoring, for determination of the safety of diagnostic tests and procedures, and for timely application of appropriate management strategies (eg, institution of prophylaxis of contrast-induced nephropathy, placement of dialysis access). GFR is widely accepted as the best indicator of renal function in both health and disease states. Accurate estimates of GFR are essential for optimizing the management of critically ill patients.

Direct measurement of GFR using urinary or plasma clearance of exogenous filtration markers (such as inulin, iothalamate, and iohexol) represents the gold standard for evaluation of renal function.[36] These tests are not routinely used in clinical practice because of high cost, low availability, and high complexity, making them highly impractical, especially in the intensive care setting. Urinary clearance of endogenous creatinine is the most-used direct measurement of GFR and can be performed in virtually every hospital laboratory. Under conditions of acute change in renal function, which is often the case in critically ill patients, 24-hour creatinine clearance (CrCl-24h) represents the most accurate estimation of renal function in the intensive care setting.[37] This cumbersome test, however, is impractical in the intensive care setting because of difficulties in obtaining accurate timed urine collections, variability in urine output, and potential inaccuracies caused by variability in creatinine generation[38] and excretion.[39] Time-limited urine collections may represent a more practical alternative in the ICU setting. In a single-center prospective study, creatinine clearance calculated based on a timed 2-hour urine collection (CrCl-2h) closely correlated with CrCl-24h (coefficient of determination $[r^2]$ = 0.88). This abbreviated creatinine clearance method was more sensitive and performed better than the Cockcroft-Gault (CG) equation or the change in the serum creatinine level in the detection of AKI (defined as CrCl-24h<60 mL/min/1.73m^2), regardless of oliguria or use of diuretics.[40] Although this method is promising, its applicability to critically ill MO individuals has not been formally evaluated.

Estimation of GFR with equations based on levels of serum creatinine and demographic and/or anthropometric data is routinely used by clinicians worldwide in daily practice. It is important to appreciate the limitations of such formulas when applying them to populations and clinical settings outside of those in which they were originally developed,[36,41] such as the MO and critically ill populations.[42] Under conditions of dynamic fluid and metabolic, hemodynamic, and hormonal changes, estimating formulas such as Modification of Diet in Renal Disease for estimating GFR (MDRD eGFR)[43] and CG creatinine clearance[44] equations should not be used to assess renal function because of the recognized inaccuracies of these equations in nonsteady states.[41,45] In fact, automated electronic eGFR (using the MDRD equation) reporting, routinely done in many institutions, may result in systematic misuse of such equations.[45]

In MO patients, physiologic changes at the level of the glomeruli and alterations of body composition bias the universal application of GFR-estimating formulas. Estimating formulas, which rely on endogenous markers to estimate renal function, are affected by generation, glomerular filtration, and tubular secretion of that specific marker (ie, serum creatinine). Overweight and obese patients have an increased GFR and renal plasma flow[16] as a maladaptive compensatory response to increased tubular reabsorption of sodium.[17] In addition, changes in body composition influence the generation of creatinine relative to measured body weight in this population. The increased body weight in the obese occurs on account of increased fat as well as lean body mass, resulting in a higher rate of creatinine generation and excretion as compared with nonobese controls.[46–48]

Several weight-based creatinine clearance–estimating formulas have been developed and evaluated in MO individuals, intending to overcome the limitations of the CG and MDRD formulas for estimating GFR (**Table 2**).[48,49] Systematic bias has been observed with all clearance equations when adjustments for body composition are not made for the obese[37] or MO populations.[48,50] For example, using measured body weight overestimates true creatinine clearance, whereas using ideal body weight underestimates true creatinine clearance with the CG equation in the MO

Table 2
Estimating creatinine clearance equations and their applicability to MO individuals

Equation (Unit)	Mathematical Formula	Original Cohort Included Obese Individuals	Validation in MO Patients
Cockcroft-Gault (mL/min)[44]	([140 − age] × weight [kg]/SCr × 72)× (0.85 if female)	No	Yes[a]
Salazar-Corcoran (mL/min)[48]	Male: (137 − age) × ([0.285 × TBW] + [12.1 × height in meters]2)/51 × SCr Female: (146 − age) × ([0.287 × TBW] + [9.74 × height in meters]2)/60 × SCr	Yes	No[b,c]
Jellife and Jellife (mL/min)[49]	(100 × weight × [F − G × (age)])/ (Scr × 1440)[c]	No	No[d]
MDRD4 (mL/min/1.73 m²)[43]	186 × SCr − 1.154 × age − 0.203 × (0.742 if female) × (1.210 if black)	No	No[e]

Abbreviations: F, 29.3 for males and 25.1 for females; G, 0.203 for males and 0.175 for females; LBW, Lean body weight; SCr, serum creatinine (in milligrams per deciliter); TBW, total body weight (kg).
 [a] Overestimated GFR when TBW used[48,50,52]; accurate when LBW used (either measured fat-free weight by bioelectric impedance analysis or calculated by the formulas of Janmahasatian and colleagues[51,52]) (LBW male = 9270 × TBW/[6680 + 216 × BMI]; LBW female = 9270 × TBW/[8780 + 244 × BMI]).[50]
 [b] Overestimated GFR in patients with BMI greater than 40.[50]
 [c] For men F = 29.3, G = 0.203 and for women F = 25.1, G = 0.175.
 [d] Overestimated GFR in patients with increasing body weight.[48]
 [e] Underestimated GFR in patients with BMI greater than 26.[42]

population.[50] Similarly, adjusted body weight, which introduces a correction factor for the difference between measured and ideal body weights in obese individuals to account for the actual increase in lean body mass of 25% to 40%, produced inaccurate results as well.[50] A mathematical model for estimation of lean body mass developed by Janmahasatian and colleagues[51] eliminated the bias introduced by the measured body weight, when used to calculate creatinine clearance by the CG formula in 8 obese patients (BMI >30).[52] Demirovic and colleagues[50] tested the accuracy of 3 equations used for estimating renal function (MDRD, CG, and the Salazar-Corcoran equations) against measured creatinine clearance with timed urine collections in 54 patients with mean a BMI of 50.5 ± 12.6. All 3 equations resulted in biased estimations of GFR. However, the use of fat-free weight (measured by electric bioimpedance) or calculated lean body weight (LBW) using the Janmahasatian formula in the CG equation resulted in clinically accurate creatinine clearance estimations.[50] These results, though promising, need to be validated in larger study populations of critically ill MO patients.

Novel serum and urinary biomarkers such as serum cystatin C, urine neutrophil gelatinase-associated lipocalin, interleukin-18, glutathione-S-transferase-p, and c-glutathione-S-transferase show promising results for early diagnosis of AKI in various clinical settings, including the ICU.[53] There are limited data on the diagnostic performance of these novel biomarkers in detecting AKI in MO individuals with or without critical illness.[54] The routine use of these biomarkers cannot be recommended at this time.

Relying on serial trends of serum creatinine levels often leads to delayed recognition of AKI because creatinine generation may be impaired in the setting of critical illness, especially sepsis.[38] Urinary flow rates, when decreasing, may offer the earliest indication of renal injury in the ICU[55] but cannot alone quantify the severity of the insult. It is not surprising that the RIFLE and AKIN criteria both include assessments of urine flow rates as part of their diagnostic and prognostic criteria.[21,22] In addition, attention to risk factors for AKI in the setting of critical illness may further improve the diagnostic sensitivity of available diagnostic tools.

While we await further studies, timed urine collections, despite their impracticalities, remain the optimal means of estimating renal function in critically ill MO patients with AKI.

CAUSES OF AKI IN THE CRITICALLY ILL MO INDIVIDUAL

The clinical approach to AKI in the critically ill MO individual follows the same general diagnostic framework as for the nonobese individual, dividing the potential causes of AKI into prerenal, renal, and obstructive categories. It is likely that the most common causes of AKI described in the nonobese critically ill patient are responsible for most cases of AKI in the MO population as well. These causes include prerenal azotemia, acute tubular necrosis (ATN), radiocontrast nephropathy, and acute interstitial nephritis. Because the general evaluation and management of these conditions have been well described elsewhere,[56,57] the authors focus the their discussion on several causes of AKI to which the MO population may be predisposed. The literature regarding specific causes of AKI in MO individuals is limited to retrospective case series and case reports (**Table 3**).

Prerenal Azotemia and ATN

Prerenal azotemia and ATN are responsible for the vast majority of cases of AKI in the ICU.[3,11,29] This finding may hold true in MO individuals, although data in this population are lacking. The most important clinical distinction between prerenal AKI and ATN is the response to intravascular fluid expansion. Improvement of renal function to baseline within 24 to 72 hours is diagnostic of prerenal disease, whereas persistent renal dysfunction in the absence of other apparent causes supports the diagnosis of ATN. At present, there are no evidence-based guidelines regarding the amount, nature, and duration of fluid resuscitation needed to effectively rule out a prerenal state.[58]

Several factors can predispose MO individuals to volume depletion and the development of AKI in the critical care setting. Overly aggressive diuresis in the setting of intravascular volume depletion (often with concomitant clinical features of volume overload, such as dependent edema), diastolic dysfunction,[59] or impaired autoregulation[32,60] may result in the development of AKI.

Intravascular volume depletion is common in the ICU setting,[61] in which factors such as critical illness, shock, malnutrition, inflammatory states, hypoalbuminemia with reduced intravascular oncotic pressure, and subsequent fluid shifts complicate the accurate assessment of intravascular volume status. Physical examination of the critically ill MO patient (in particular, the estimation of central venous pressure by jugular venous pressure measurement on clinical examination) can be misleading.[62] Obesity can be associated with edema, independent of the presence of fluid overload.[63] Decisions regarding volume management either by aggressive administration of intravenous fluids or by volume removal via the administration of diuretics or ultrafiltration, based solely on the presence of peripheral edema in this population, may lead to serious consequences such as fluid overload with worsening of interstitial and pulmonary edema, hemodynamic compromise with potential exacerbation of the renal injury, or eventually increased morbidity and mortality.[64,65] Given

Table 3
Causes of AKI in MO patients reported in the literature

Investigators	Cause	Number of Cases Reported	Acute Renal Support Requirement	Outcomes
Sharma et al,[32] 2006 Pasnik et al,[85] 2005 Sakpal et al,[107] 2009 Friedman et al,[103] 2008 Caruso et al, 1998[104]	AKI in the setting of multiple organ failure	13	Yes in 2 patients Not reported in 11	1 patient deceased[103] 1 patient with complete resolution of AKI[104] Not reported in 11
Nasr et al,[69] 2008 Nelson et al,[108] 2005	Acute oxalate nephropathy after bariatric surgery	10	7	7 patients progressed to ESRD 3 patients developed stage 3–4 CKD
Courtney et al,[77] 2007 Singh et al,[76] 2007 Karamadoukis et al,[78] 2009	Acute oxalate nephropathy associated with orlistat therapy	3	2	2 patients developed ESRD[69] 1 patient with partial resolution of AKI with discontinuation of drug and hydration[77]
Bostanjian et al,[81] 2003 Collier et al,[82] 2003 Goyal and Goyal,[83] 1998 Guzzi et al,[84] 1993 Pasnik et al,[85] 2005 Roth,[86] 2007 Torres-Villalobos et al,[87] 2003	Pigment nephropathy in the setting of rhabdomyolysis	10	7	4 patients deceased[81,82] 3 patients with complete resolution of AKI[81,85,87] 1 patient with partial resolution of AKI[83] In 2 patients, renal outcomes were not reported[84,86]
Rhodes et al,[109] 1979	Intra-abdominal hypertension, ACS	1	No	Resolution of AKI with change in position
Panner et al,[110] 1970	Fluoride nephrotoxicity after methoxyflurane anesthesia	1	NA	Deceased
Asim and Turney,[111] 1996 Winn et al,[112] 1997	Intermittent ureteric obstruction[113]	2	No	Improvement after ureteric stenting[111] and surgical correction of abdominal hernia[112]
Korzets et al,[114] 1998 Alsina et al,[115] 2009	Renal AA amyloidosis	2	No	Deceased[114] Not reported[115]
Nair and Said,[116] 2005	Anti-GBM disease	1	Not reported	Not reported
Soto et al,[117] 2005	IgA nephropathy	1	Temporary	Improvement of AKI after bariatric surgery

Abbreviations: AA, amyloid A; ACS, abdominal compartment syndrome; GBM, glomerular basement membrane; ESRD, end-stage renal disease; NA, not available.

the inherent challenges associated with accurately determining the intravascular volume status in the critically ill MO individual, invasive hemodynamic monitoring may offer valuable additional information to provide specific therapeutic goals.[65,66]

A thorough history can uncover important clues regarding the intravascular volume status of a patient, such as extrarenal loss of volume (fever, prolonged fasting, vomiting, diarrhea, bleeding), presence of third spacing (low oncotic pressure states, pancreatitis, burns, and so forth), diminished cardiac output (cardiomyopathy, acute coronary syndromes, pericardial disease), and the presence of shock. The urine sediment is usually bland in prerenal azotemia as opposed to other pathologic processes in which muddy brown casts (ATN) and sterile pyuria and white blood cell casts (interstitial nephritis) may be seen. A low fractional excretion of sodium (<1.0%) suggests volume depletion with a relatively intact tubular reabsorptive capacity, thus assisting in the differentiation of prerenal azotemia from ATN.[56] It is important to recognize that the test may be falsely elevated in the setting of diuretic therapy, and the fractional excretion of urea may better discriminate between reversible prerenal azotemia and ATN in this setting.[67] In addition, careful review of the urinary flow rates can be helpful in distinguishing prerenal azotemia from ATN: oliguria is less common with prerenal azotemia and anuria is distinctly uncommon in cases of prerenal azotemia.

Early differentiation of prerenal azotemia and ATN is important because a diagnosis of ATN will help minimize overaggressive resuscitation efforts, which in turn may impair hemodynamics and wound healing.[68]

Acute Oxalate Nephropathy

Acute oxalate nephropathy is a type of ATN caused by direct precipitation of oxalate in the renal tubules, causing acute obstruction and tubular injury. Several investigators have reported the occurrence of hyperoxaluria, hyperoxaluric nephrolithiasis, and acute oxalate nephropathy in MO individuals after bariatric surgery.[69–75] Cases of severe renal injury with biopsy-proven acute oxalate nephropathy were initially reported in patients who underwent jejunoileal bypass.[71,74] This procedure has been abandoned due to high rates of complications such as liver failure, electrolyte imbalances, diarrhea, nephrolithiasis, oxalate nephropathy, and death.[72] Data are emerging on the complications of enteral hyperoxaluria (nephrolithiasis and acute or chronic oxalate nephropathy) and modern gastric bypass procedures.[69,70]

Orlistat, a gastrointestinal lipase inhibitor commonly used for weight reduction in obese patients, has recently been reported to cause acute oxalate nephropathy in obese patients with or without underlying CKD.[76–78] In these patients, AKI was temporally associated with orlistat therapy and development of fat malabsorption. End-stage renal disease occurred in most patients.[69,78] Of note, in one case the AKI proved partially reversible after discontinuation of the drug and hydration, with resolution of tubular oxalate crystal deposition observed in a kidney biopsy 1 month later.[77]

The mechanism of enteric hyperoxaluria induced by orlistat or seen after bariatric surgery is fat malabsorption. This mechanism has been demonstrated in an animal model of obesity in adult rats.[79] In normal subjects, dietary oxalate complexes with calcium, forming insoluble salts that are eventually excreted in feces. Fat malabsorption results in chelation of calcium by free fatty acids, thus increasing the unbound fraction of oxalate in the intestinal lumen available for absorption.[70] In addition, the increased load of fatty acids in intestinal contents may increase the colonic permeability, allowing for increased oxalate absorption in the colon.[80]

Urine sediment analysis in patients developing acute oxalate nephropathy reveals many calcium oxalate crystals, and 24-hour urine collections demonstrate marked hyperoxaluria.[69] On renal biopsy, pathognomonic changes consisting of calcium oxalate crystal deposition in tubular lumens can be seen.[69,74]

Rhabdomyolysis and Pigment Nephropathy

MO patients undergoing bariatric surgery are at higher risk of pressure-induced rhabdomyolysis.[81–87] In a case-control study of 6 MO individuals who underwent a duodenal switch procedure and developed postoperative rhabdomyolysis, Bostanjian and colleagues[81] reported that 3 of 6 patients developed severe AKI, requiring dialysis; all patients eventually died. Of the remaining survivors, 1 of the 3 developed reversible AKI. Increases in median creatinine phosphokinase levels in affected patients ranged from 26,000 to 29,000 IU/L versus 1200 IU/L in controls. All patients who developed rhabdomyolysis presented with an area of an early decubitus skin ulcer in the buttock and eventually developed extensive myonecrosis of the medial gluteal muscles, requiring extensive debridement. These patients had a higher BMI (median 67) compared with controls (median BMI 55) and a higher operative time (median of 5.7 hours) compared with controls (median 4.0 hours, $P = .01$).[81] MO patients who undergo prolonged surgeries, in whom physical examination is difficult, who have low intravascular volume status despite presence of pitting edema, and who have higher BMI appear to be at higher risk of rhabdomyolysis-induced AKI.[82] In addition, an exaggerated lithotomy position may predispose a person to rhabdomyolysis and AKI.[84,86]

Attention to intraoperative padding and positioning, limiting the duration of surgery, and rigorous attention to skin care and surveillance may help prevent pressure myonecrosis, rhabdomyolysis, and subsequent pigment nephropathy. These measures should be routinely instituted in critically ill MO patients. Postoperative prophylactic measures should include routine postoperative creatine kinase measurements, attention to volume status, and early correction of intravascular depletion with isotonic fluids.[81] The general principles of management of rhabdomyolysis–induced renal injury apply in the MO critically ill patient, and these principles have been the subject of review.[88]

Intra-Abdominal Hypertension and Abdominal Compartment Syndrome

Intra-abdominal hypertension (IAH) and abdominal compartment syndrome (ACS) represent common causes of AKI in the critical care setting and have emerged as important predictors of morbidity and mortality in the general population of critically ill patients.[89–91] IAH is defined as an intra-abdominal pressure (IAP) greater than 12 mm Hg on 3 measurements obtained 4 to 6 hours apart.[92,93] IAH can lead to ACS, defined as IAP greater than 20 mm Hg, with or without an abdominal perfusion pressure (ie, the difference between mean arterial pressure and the IAP) less than 60 mm Hg on 2 measurements obtained 1 to 6 hours apart, associated with a single- or multiple-organ system failure that was not previously present.[92] Indirect transduction of the urinary bladder via balloon catheter is the most commonly used method for determining IAP because of its simplicity and minimal cost, and the technique of IAP measurements has recently been standardized.[92]

ACS is characterized clinically by multiorgan dysfunction, including oliguric or anuric AKI, low cardiac output caused by impaired venous return and increased afterload, decreased respiratory system compliance, intracranial pressure elevation, hypotension, and metabolic acidosis. The mechanisms of oliguria include increased renal vascular resistance and increased intraparenchymal renal pressures.[94] IAH is an independent predictor of AKI in the intensive care setting.[90] Generic causes of IAH and ACS are ascites, hemorrhage or visceral organ edema in trauma patients, pancreatitis, massive hemorrhage, ileus, and overly vigorous fluid resuscitation with third spacing.[94] Unfortunately, there are no studies evaluating the epidemiology of ACS or IAP in critically ill MO individuals. However, certain physiologic characteristics may place this population at risk of developing ACS; IAPs and BMI are positively correlated, and obese individuals have higher IAP than nonobese controls.[95] Abdominal decompression is the mainstay of therapy for IAH, often necessitating decompressive laparotomy, paracentesis, and/or aggressive management of ileus.[94]

Peritoneal gas insufflation used in laparoscopic surgery is associated with increased vascular resistance, decreased cardiac index, transient oliguria, and a case of reversible oliguric AKI in a nonobese patient.[96] A 64% relative decrease in the intraoperative urine output has been observed in MO patients undergoing laparoscopic Roux-en-Y gastric bypass compared with similar patients who underwent the open procedure[97]; however, no significant changes in blood urea nitrogen or serum creatinine levels were observed in the perioperative period after laparoscopic gastric bypass.[98] Whether peritoneal gas insufflation is a risk factor for postoperative AKI in MO individuals undergoing laparoscopic procedures is not known.

The contribution of increased abdominal pressure to cases of postoperative AKI or AKI in the ICU setting in MO individuals is not clear, and further research is warranted.

RENAL SUPPORT IN CRITICALLY ILL OBESE PATIENTS

In the absence of effective pharmacologic therapies for AKI in critically ill patients, management is supportive and aimed at reversing potential causative factors, such as sepsis, hypotension, urinary tract obstruction, among others. Appropriate attention to nutritional support and medication dose adjustments are integral components of the management of the MO patients with AKI. In severe cases of acute renal injury, RRT is a central component of this supportive care. The goals of RRT in the ICU include effective clearance of uremic toxins, optimization of volume status, and management of acid-base and electrolyte disturbances. Data from the Project to Improve Care in Acute Renal Disease (PICARD) cohort would suggest that more than half of the patients with AKI in the critical care setting may require RRT and a large proportion will do so concurrent with hemodynamic instability.[11] Because of the uncertainty of available evidence, the optimal timing, dose, and modality of RRT in critically ill individuals remain in question.[99-101] Clinical practice patterns are often subject to resource availability and individual physician preferences rather than evidence-based guidelines.[101,102] These gaps in knowledge apply equally to the MO critically ill population, because there are no reported observational or randomized controlled trials examining these important issues in this population.

The literature regarding RRT in critically ill MO patients is limited to 2 case reports.[103,104] In the first case, a 466-kg man with sepsis and cocaine-induced lung injury underwent continuous venovenous hemofiltration (CVVH) for oligoanuric AKI. CVVH was used initially because of specific hospital plumbing issues, limiting the use of dialysis-based modalities in that specific location. Therapy was initiated via a temporary 19.5-cm dialysis catheter inserted at the bedside under ultrasonographic guidance in the right internal jugular vein without radiological confirmation of adequate placement. Before access placement, an industrial-grade lift was used to position the patient. Assessments of volume status, dialysis dose, and medication dosing were based on trial and error. CVVH was initiated with 6 L of replacement fluid hourly. An actual weight-based CVVH dosing of 35 mL/kg/min in the general ICU population has been found to be associated with better outcomes as opposed to a lower dose of 20 mL/kg/min.[105] In this case, the 35-mL/kg/min dose would have resulted in the

> **Box 1**
> **Proposed areas of research needed in the MO critically ill patient**
>
> Is AKI incidence (and causes) in MO different from that in the nonobese crucially ill population?
>
> What are the outcomes of MO critically ill patients who develop AKI?
>
> What are the optimal ways of assessing renal function in the critically ill MO patient?
>
> What is the performance of novel biomarkers of AKI in the critically ill MO patient?
>
> What is the optimal management strategy (timing, dosing, and modality) for RRTs in the MO critically ill patient?

need for 16 L/h of replacement fluids, a volume which may prove impractical for the pharmaceutical team to support. Conventional dialysis was performed when room plumbing was modified. The patient then underwent daily treatments for 4 to 6 hours with a high-flux membrane. Despite adequate achievement of fluid and metabolic control, care was withdrawn due to progressive complications of sepsis.[103]

The second reported case was that of a 54-year-old MO woman (BMI not reported) who developed AKI in the setting of a spontaneous cerebellar hemorrhage. CVVH was chosen as the modality of choice with the goal of preventing significant fluctuations in the intracranial pressure. Dialysate solution was delivered at 1500 to 1600 mL/h, with a net ultrafiltration of 600 to 1200 mL/h. With intensive supportive care, the patient made a full neurologic and renal recovery.[104]

These cases illustrate the challenges specific to this population. Vascular access is often difficult to obtain safely in critically ill MO patients. There is loss of anatomic landmarks from excess adipose tissue, and imaging studies are also limited in their ability to be interpreted.[62] Use of bedside ultrasonographic techniques for temporary vascular access and interventional radiology services can be of great value in establishing prompt vascular access safely.[103] Several aspects of RRT in critically ill MO patients deserve further mention. Dosing continuous therapies based on actual weight can result in the requirement of impractical and massive volume of replacement fluid. Although the optimal dosing of continuous RRTs in the general critically ill population is not well understood, this issue may be even more important in the MO patients from a practical standpoint. Alterations in body composition may play a significant role in the special RRT needs in this population, and estimated or direct LBW adjustments may result in a more suitable RRT prescription.

Logistic issues related to the effective delivery of RRT to critically ill MO patients include transportation (special bariatric ambulances can carry up to 455 kg[106]) and the critical care unit infrastructure, which often can be challenged by the care of an MO patient. It is important for emergency preparedness of health care facilities, dialysis staff, and ICUs to take such factors into consideration well in advance when delivering RRT to this special population.

SUMMARY

AKI in critically ill MO patients poses significant challenges in diagnosis and management for practicing clinicians. The available body of literature suggests that AKI is not uncommon in this population; however, information regarding the effect of morbid obesity on adverse outcomes in critically ill patients with AKI remains unanswered. Other unexplored areas are highlighted in **Box 1**. Knowledge of these areas should help us better understand the epidemiology, causes, risk factors, and optimal management strategies for critically ill MO individuals with AKI. Further research exploring the spectrum of acute renal disease in this challenging and prevalent population is critically needed.

REFERENCES

1. U.S. Renal Data System. USRDS 2009 annual data report: atlas of end-stage renal disease in the United States. Bethesda (MD): National Institutes of Health, National Institute of Diabetes and Digestive and Kidney Diseases; 2009.
2. Waikar SS, Wald R, Chertow GM, et al. Validity of international classification of diseases, ninth revision, clinical modification codes for acute renal failure. J Am Soc Nephrol 2006;17(6):1688–94.
3. Uchino S, Kellum JA, Bellomo R, et al. Beginning and Ending Supportive Therapy for the Kidney (BEST Kidney) Investigators. Acute renal failure in critically ill patients: a multinational, multicenter study. JAMA 2005;294(7):813–8.
4. Akinnusi ME, Pineda LA, El Solh AA. Effect of obesity on intensive care morbidity and mortality: a meta-analysis. Crit Care Med 2008;36(1):151–8 [see comment].
5. Nasraway SA Jr, Albert M, Donnelly AM, et al. Morbid obesity is an independent determinant of death among surgical critically ill patients. Crit Care Med 2006; 34(4):964–70.
6. Waikar SS, Liu KD, Chertow GM. Diagnosis, epidemiology and outcomes of acute kidney injury. Clin J Am Soc Nephrol 2008;3(3):844–61.
7. Vandijck DM, Oeyen S, Decruyenaere JM, et al. Acute kidney injury, length of stay, and costs in patients hospitalized in the intensive care unit. Acta Clin Belg Suppl 2007;2:341–5.
8. Tsagalis G, Akrivos T, Alevizaki M, et al. Long-term prognosis of acute kidney injury after first acute stroke. Clin J Am Soc Nephrol 2009;4(3):616–22.
9. Hsu C, Chertow GM, McCulloch CE, et al. Nonrecovery of kidney function and death after acute on chronic renal failure. Clin J Am Soc Nephrol 2009;4(5): 891–8.
10. Hoste EA, Clermont G, Kersten A, et al. RIFLE criteria for acute kidney injury are associated with hospital mortality in critically ill patients: a cohort analysis. Crit Care 2006;10(3):R73.
11. Mehta RL, Pascual MT, Soroko S, et al. Spectrum of acute renal failure in the intensive care unit: the PICARD experience. Kidney Int 2004;66(4):1613–21.
12. Elsayed EF, Sarnak MJ, Tighiouart H, et al. Waist-to-hip ratio, body mass index, and subsequent kidney disease and death. Am J Kidney Dis 2008;52(1):29–38.
13. Foster MC, Hwang SJ, Larson MG, et al. Overweight, obesity, and the development of stage 3 CKD: the Framingham Heart Study. Am J Kidney Dis 2008;52(1): 39–48.
14. Ross WR, McGill JB. Epidemiology of obesity and chronic kidney disease. Adv Chronic Kidney Dis 2006;13(4):325–35.
15. Hoste EA, Kellum JA. Acute kidney injury: epidemiology and diagnostic criteria. Curr Opin Crit Care 2006;12(6):531–7.
16. Chagnac A, Weinstein T, Korzets A, et al. Glomerular hemodynamics in severe obesity. Am J Physiol Renal Physiol 2000;278(5):F817–22.
17. Chagnac A, Herman M, Zingerman B, et al. Obesity-induced glomerular hyperfiltration: its involvement in the pathogenesis of tubular sodium reabsorption. Nephrol Dial Transplant 2008;23(12):3946–52.
18. Kambham N, Markowitz GS, Valeri AM, et al. Obesity-related glomerulopathy: an emerging epidemic. Kidney Int 2001;59(4):1498–509.

19. Uchino S, Bellomo R, Goldsmith D, et al. An assessment of the RIFLE criteria for acute renal failure in hospitalized patients. Crit Care Med 2006;34(7):1913–7.

20. Chertow GM, Burdick E, Honour M, et al. Acute kidney injury, mortality, length of stay, and costs in hospitalized patients. J Am Soc Nephrol 2005;16(11): 3365–70.

21. Mehta RL, Kellum JA, Shah SV, et al. Acute kidney injury network: report of an initiative to improve outcomes in acute kidney injury. Crit Care 2007;11(2):R31.

22. Bellomo R, Ronco C, Kellum JA, et al. Acute Dialysis Quality Initiative Workgroup. Acute renal failure—definition, outcome measures, animal models, fluid therapy and information technology needs: the second international consensus conference of the acute dialysis quality initiative (ADQI) group. Crit Care 2004;8(4):R204–12 [see comment].

23. Uchino S, Bellomo R, Morimatsu H, et al. Continuous renal replacement therapy: a worldwide practice survey. The beginning and ending supportive therapy for the kidney (B.E.S.T. kidney) investigators. Intensive Care Med 2007;33(9): 1563–70.

24. Peake SL, Moran JL, Ghelani DR, et al. The effect of obesity on 12-month survival following admission to intensive care: a prospective study. Crit Care Med 2006;34(12):2929–39.

25. Hoste EA, Schurgers M. Epidemiology of acute kidney injury: how big is the problem? Crit Care Med 2008;36(4 Suppl):S146–51.

26. Ali T, Khan I, Simpson W, et al. Incidence and outcomes in acute kidney injury: a comprehensive population-based study. J Am Soc Nephrol 2007;18(4): 1292–8.

27. Joannidis M, Metnitz B, Bauer P, et al. Acute kidney injury in critically ill patients classified by AKIN versus RIFLE using the SAPS 3 database. Intensive Care Med 2009;35(10):1692–702.

28. Joffe A, Wood K. Obesity in critical care. Curr Opin Anaesthesiol 2007;20(2): 113–8.

29. Hoste EA, De Corte W. Epidemiology of AKI in the ICU. Acta Clin Belg Suppl 2007;2:314–7.

30. Bagshaw SM, George C, Bellomo R, ANZICS Database Management Committe. A comparison of the RIFLE and AKIN criteria for acute kidney injury in critically ill patients. Nephrol Dial Transplant 2008;23(5):1569–74.

31. McCullough PA, Gallagher MJ, Dejong AT, et al. Cardiorespiratory fitness and short-term complications after bariatric surgery. Chest 2006;130(2):517–25.

32. Sharma SK, McCauley J, Cottam D, et al. Acute changes in renal function after laparoscopic gastric surgery for morbid obesity. Surg Obes Relat Dis 2006;2(3): 389–92.

33. Thakar CV, Kharat V, Blanck S, et al. Acute kidney injury after gastric bypass surgery. Clin J Am Soc Nephrol 2007;2(3):426–30.

34. Wigfield CH, Lindsey JD, Munoz A, et al. Is extreme obesity a risk factor for cardiac surgery? An analysis of patients with a BMI > or = 40. Eur J Cardiothorac Surg 2006;29(4):434–40.

35. Yap CH, Mohajeri M, Yii M. Obesity and early complications after cardiac surgery. Med J Aust 2007;186(7):350–4.

36. Stevens LA, Levey AS. Measured GFR as a confirmatory test for estimated GFR. J Am Soc Nephrol 2009;20(11):2305–13.

37. Snider RD, Kruse JA, Bander JJ, et al. Accuracy of estimated creatinine clearance in obese patients with stable renal function in the intensive care unit. Pharmacotherapy 1995;15(6):747–53.

38. Doi K, Yuen PS, Eisner C, et al. Reduced production of creatinine limits its use as marker of kidney injury in sepsis. J Am Soc Nephrol 2009;20(6):1217–21.
39. Jacobi D, Lavigne C, Halimi JM, et al. Variability in creatinine excretion in adult diabetic, overweight men and women: consequences on creatinine-based classification of renal disease. Diabetes Res Clin Pract 2008;80(1):102–7.
40. Herrera-Gutierrez ME, Seller-Perez G, Banderas-Bravo E, et al. Replacement of 24-h creatinine clearance by 2-h creatinine clearance in intensive care unit patients: a single-center study. Intensive Care Med 2007;33(11):1900–6.
41. Stevens LA, Coresh J, Greene T, et al. Assessing kidney function—measured and estimated glomerular filtration rate. N Engl J Med 2006;354(23):2473–83.
42. Stevens LA, Coresh J, Feldman HI, et al. Evaluation of the modification of diet in renal disease study equation in a large diverse population. J Am Soc Nephrol 2007;18(10):2749–57.
43. Levey AS, Bosch JP, Lewis JB, et al. A more accurate method to estimate glomerular filtration rate from serum creatinine: a new prediction equation. Modification of Diet in Renal Disease Study Group. Ann Intern Med 1999;130(6):461–70.
44. Cockcroft DW, Gault MH. Prediction of creatinine clearance from serum creatinine. Nephron 1976;16(1):31–41.
45. Nguyen MT, Maynard SE, Kimmel PL. Misapplications of commonly used kidney equations: renal physiology in practice. Clin J Am Soc Nephrol 2009;4(3):528–34.
46. Tager BN, Kirsch HW. Creatinine excretion in women: clinical significance in obesity. J Clin Endocrinol 1942;2(12):696–9.
47. Smith OW. Creatinine excretion in women: data collected in the course of urinalysis for female sex hormones. J Clin Endocrinol 1942;2(1):1–12.
48. Salazar DE, Corcoran GB. Predicting creatinine clearance and renal drug clearance in obese patients from estimated fat-free body mass. Am J Med 1988;84(6):1053–60.
49. Jelliffe RW, Jelliffe SM. Estimation of creatinine clearance from changing serum-creatinine levels. Lancet 1971;2(7726):710.
50. Demirovic JA, Pai AB, Pai MP. Estimation of creatinine clearance in morbidly obese patients. Am J Health Syst Pharm 2009;66(7):642–8.
51. Janmahasatian S, Duffull SB, Ash S, et al. Quantification of lean bodyweight. Clin Pharmacokinet 2005;44(10):1051–65.
52. Janmahasatian S, Duffull SB, Chagnac A, et al. Lean body mass normalizes the effect of obesity on renal function. Br J Clin Pharmacol 2008;65(6):964–5.
53. Coca SG, Yalavarthy R, Concato J, et al. Biomarkers for the diagnosis and risk stratification of acute kidney injury: a systematic review. Kidney Int 2008;73(9):1008–16.
54. Schuck O, Teplan V, Stollova M, et al. Estimation of glomerular filtration rate in obese patients with chronic renal impairment based on serum cystatin C levels. Clin Nephrol 2004;62(2):92–6.
55. Macedo E, Malhotra R, Bouchard J, et al. Do episodes of oliguria reflect acute kidney injury in critically ill patients? J Am Soc Nephrol 2009;20:115A.
56. Lameire N, Van Biesen W, Vanholder R. Acute renal failure. Lancet 2005;365 (9457):417–30.
57. Dennen P, Douglas IS, Anderson R. Acute kidney injury in the intensive care unit: an update and primer for the intensivist. Crit Care Med 2010;38(1):261–75.
58. Macedo E, Mehta RL. Prerenal failure: from old concepts to new paradigms. Curr Opin Crit Care 2009;15(6):467–73.

59. Pilz B, Brasen JH, Schneider W, et al. Obesity and hypertension-induced restrictive cardiomyopathy: a harbinger of things to come. Hypertension 2004;43(5): 911–7.
60. Blantz RC. Pathophysiology of pre-renal azotemia. Kidney Int 1998;53(2): 512–23.
61. Finfer S, Bellomo R, Boyce N, et al. A comparison of albumin and saline for fluid resuscitation in the intensive care unit. N Engl J Med 2004;350(22):2247–56.
62. El-Solh AA. Clinical approach to the critically ill, morbidly obese patient. Am J Respir Crit Care Med 2004;169(5):557–61 [see comment].
63. Agarwal R, Andersen MJ, Pratt JH. On the importance of pedal edema in hemodialysis patients. Clin J Am Soc Nephrol 2008;3(1):153–8.
64. van der Heijden M, Verheij J, van Nieuw Amerongen GP, et al. Crystalloid or colloid fluid loading and pulmonary permeability, edema, and injury in septic and nonseptic critically ill patients with hypovolemia. Crit Care Med 2009;37 (4):1275–81.
65. Murphy CV, Schramm GE, Doherty JA, et al. The importance of fluid management in acute lung injury secondary to septic shock. Chest 2009;136(1): 102–9.
66. Rivers EP, Nguyen HB, Huang DT, et al. Early goal-directed therapy. Crit Care Med 2004;32(1):314–5.
67. Carvounis CP, Nisar S, Guro-Razuman S. Significance of the fractional excretion of urea in the differential diagnosis of acute renal failure. Kidney Int 2002;62(6): 2223–9.
68. Prowle JR, Echeverri JE, Ligabo E, et al. Fluid balance and acute kidney injury. Nat Rev Nephrol 2010;6(2):107–15.
69. Nasr SH, D'Agati VD, Said SM, et al. Oxalate nephropathy complicating Roux-en-Y gastric bypass: an underrecognized cause of irreversible renal failure. Clin J Am Soc Nephrol 2008;3(6):1676–83.
70. Asplin JR, Coe FL. Hyperoxaluria in kidney stone formers treated with modern bariatric surgery. J Urol 2007;177(2):565–9.
71. Hassan I, Juncos LA, Milliner DS, et al. Chronic renal failure secondary to oxalate nephropathy: a preventable complication after jejunoileal bypass. Mayo Clin Proc 2001;76(7):758–60.
72. Requarth JA, Burchard KW, Colacchio TA, et al. Long-term morbidity following jejunoileal bypass. The continuing potential need for surgical reversal. Arch Surg 1995;130(3):318–25.
73. Sinha MK, Collazo-Clavell ML, Rule A, et al. Hyperoxaluric nephrolithiasis is a complication of Roux-en-Y gastric bypass surgery. Kidney Int 2007;72(1): 100–7.
74. Mole DR, Tomson CR, Mortensen N, et al. Renal complications of jejuno-ileal bypass for obesity. QJM 2001;94(2):69–77.
75. Ehlers SM, Posalaky Z, Strate RG, et al. Acute reversible renal failure following jejunoileal bypass for morbid obesity: a clinical and pathological (EM) study of a case. Surgery 1977;82(5):629–34.
76. Singh A, Sarkar SR, Gaber LW, et al. Acute oxalate nephropathy associated with orlistat, a gastrointestinal lipase inhibitor. Am J Kidney Dis 2007;49(1):153–7.
77. Courtney AE, O'Rourke DM, Maxwell AP. Rapidly progressive renal failure associated with successful pharmacotherapy for obesity. Nephrol Dial Transplant 2007;22(2):621–3.
78. Karamadoukis L, Shivashankar GH, Ludeman L, et al. An unusual complication of treatment with orlistat. Clin Nephrol 2009;71(4):430–2.

79. Ferraz RR, Tiselius HG, Heilberg IP. Fat malabsorption induced by gastrointestinal lipase inhibitor leads to an increase in urinary oxalate excretion. Kidney Int 2004;66(2):676–82.
80. Dobbins JW, Binder HJ. Importance of the colon in enteric hyperoxaluria. N Engl J Med 1977;296(6):298–301.
81. Bostanjian D, Anthone GJ, Hamoui N, et al. Rhabdomyolysis of gluteal muscles leading to renal failure: a potentially fatal complication of surgery in the morbidly obese. Obes Surg 2003;13(2):302–5.
82. Collier B, Goreja MA, Duke BE 3rd. Postoperative rhabdomyolysis with bariatric surgery. Obes Surg 2003;13(6):941–3.
83. Goyal SB, Goyal RS. Diabetic ketoacidosis and rhabdomyolysis following excessive intake of a weight reducing diet. Ren Fail 1998;20(4):645–7.
84. Guzzi LM, Mills LM, Greenman P. Rhabdomyolysis, acute renal failure, and the exaggerated lithotomy position. Anesth Analg 1993;77(3):635–7.
85. Pasnik K, Krupa J, Stanowski E, et al. Successful treatment of gastric fistula following rhabdomyolysis after vertical banded gastroplasty. Obes Surg 2005; 15(3):428–30.
86. Roth JV. Bilateral sciatic and femoral neuropathies, rhabdomyolysis, and acute renal failure caused by positioning during radical retropubic prostatectomy. Anesth Analg 2007;105(6):1747–8.
87. Torres-Villalobos G, Kimura E, Mosqueda JL, et al. Pressure-induced rhabdomyolysis after bariatric surgery. Obes Surg 2003;13(2):297–301.
88. Bosch X, Poch E, Grau JM. Rhabdomyolysis and acute kidney injury. N Engl J Med 2009;361(1):62–72.
89. Shibagaki Y, Tai C, Nayak A, et al. Intra-abdominal hypertension is an underappreciated cause of acute renal failure. Nephrol Dial Transplant 2006;21(12): 3567–70.
90. Dalfino L, Tullo L, Donadio I, et al. Intra-abdominal hypertension and acute renal failure in critically ill patients. Intensive Care Med 2008;34(4):707–13.
91. Sugrue M, Balogh Z, Malbrain M. Intra-abdominal hypertension and renal failure. ANZ J Surg 2004;74(1–2):78.
92. Malbrain ML, Cheatham ML, Kirkpatrick A, et al. Results from the international conference of experts on intra-abdominal hypertension and abdominal compartment syndrome. I. Definitions. Intensive Care Med 2006;32(11):1722–32.
93. Cheatham ML, Malbrain ML, Kirkpatrick A, et al. Results from the international conference of experts on intra-abdominal hypertension and abdominal compartment syndrome. II. Recommendations. Intensive Care Med 2007; 33(6):951–62.
94. Sugrue M. Abdominal compartment syndrome. Curr Opin Crit Care 2005;11(4): 333–8.
95. Lambert DM, Marceau S, Forse RA. Intra-abdominal pressure in the morbidly obese. Obes Surg 2005;15(9):1225–32.
96. Ben-David B, Croitoru M, Gaitini L. Acute renal failure following laparoscopic cholecystectomy: a case report. J Clin Anesth 1999;11(6):486–9.
97. Nguyen NT, Wolfe BM. The physiologic effects of pneumoperitoneum in the morbidly obese. Ann Surg 2005;241(2):219–26.
98. Nguyen NT, Perez RV, Fleming N, et al. Effect of prolonged pneumoperitoneum on intraoperative urine output during laparoscopic gastric bypass. J Am Coll Surg 2002;195(4):476–83.
99. Seabra VF, Balk EM, Liangos O, et al. Timing of renal replacement therapy initiation in acute renal failure: a meta-analysis. Am J Kidney Dis 2008;52(2):272–84.

100. VA/NIH Acute Renal Failure Trial Network, Palevsky PM, Zhang JH, O'Connor TZ, et al. Intensity of renal support in critically ill patients with acute kidney injury. N Engl J Med 2008;359(1):7–20.

101. Overberger P, Pesacreta M, Palevsky PM, VA/NIH Acute Renal Failure Trial Network. Management of renal replacement therapy in acute kidney injury: a survey of practitioner prescribing practices. Clin J Am Soc Nephrol 2007; 2(4):623–30.

102. Gatward JJ, Gibbon GJ, Wrathall G, et al. Renal replacement therapy for acute renal failure: a survey of practice in adult intensive care units in the united kingdom. Anaesthesia 2008;63(9):959–66.

103. Friedman AN, Decker B, Seele L, et al. Challenges of treating a 466-kilogram man with acute kidney injury. Am J Kidney Dis 2008;52(1):140–3.

104. Caruso DM, Vishteh AG, Greene KA, et al. Continuous hemodialysis for the management of acute renal failure in the presence of cerebellar hemorrhage. Case report. J Neurosurg 1998;89(4):649–52.

105. Ronco C, Bellomo R, Homel P, et al. Effects of different doses in continuous veno-venous haemofiltration on outcomes of acute renal failure: a prospective randomised trial. Lancet 2000;356(9223):26–30.

106. Berger E. Emergency departments shoulder challenges of providing care, preserving dignity for the "super obese". Ann Emerg Med 2007;50(4):443–5.

107. Sakpal SV, Patel C, Chamberlain RS. Near lethal endometriosis and a massive (64 kg) endometrioma: case report and review of the literature. Clin Exp Obstet Gynecol 2009;36(1):49–52.

108. Nelson WK, Houghton SG, Milliner DS, et al. Enteric hyperoxaluria, nephrolithiasis, and oxalate nephropathy: Potentially serious and unappreciated complications of Roux-en-Y gastric bypass. Surg Obes Relat Dis 2005;1(5):481–5.

109. Rhodes JM, Graham-Brown RA, Sarkany I. Reversible renal failure in an obese patient: hazard of sitting with feet continuously elevated. Lancet 1979;2(8133):96.

110. Panner BJ, Freeman RB, Roth-Moyo LA, et al. Toxicity following methoxyflurane anesthesia. I. Clinical and pathological observations in two fatal cases. JAMA 1970;214(1):86–90.

111. Asim M, Turney JH. Intermittent ureteric obstruction caused by 'floating' renal transplant. Nephrol Dial Transplant 1996;11(8):1637–8.

112. Winn MP, Bollinger RR, Conlon PJ. Orthostatic acute renal failure in a renal transplant. Transpl Int 1997;10(5):395–7.

113. Mianné D, Dessart P, Lanfrey P, et al. [Acute obstructive renal failure and scrotal complete hernia of the bladder. apropos of a case, review of the literature]. J Chir (Paris) 1996;133(9–10):459–61 [in French].

114. Korzets Z, Smorjik Y, Zahavi T, et al. Renal AA amyloidosis—a long-term sequela of jejuno-ileal bypass. Nephrol Dial Transplant 1998;13(7):1843–5.

115. Alsina E, Martin M, Panades M, et al. Renal AA amyloidosis secondary to morbid obesity? Clin Nephrol 2009;72(4):312–4.

116. Nair R, Said M. Diabetic woman with massive proteinuria and acute renal failure. Am J Kidney Dis 2005;46(2):362–6.

117. Soto FC, Higa-Sansone G, Copley JB, et al. Renal failure, glomerulonephritis and morbid obesity: improvement after rapid weight loss following laparoscopic gastric bypass. Obes Surg 2005;15(1):137–40.

Gastrointestinal System and Obesity

Doyle D. Ashburn, DO[a], Mary Jane Reed, MD, FCCM, FCCP[b],*

KEYWORDS

- Gastrointestinal • Obesity • GERD • NASH
- Abdominal compartment syndrome

Several significant changes occur in the gastrointestinal system with obesity that can effect management in critical illness. This population is at risk for gastroesophageal reflux disease (GERD), abdominal compartment syndrome, nonalcoholic fatty liver disease (NAFLD), and an increased incidence of cholelithiasis. It is important for critical care providers to be aware of these potential complicating factors.

An increase in the prevalence of GERD and obesity has occurred in recent years, and this confluence of the two epidemics has generated great interest in the association between the disorders.[1] Several studies within the past decade have shown a relationship between increased body mass index (BMI) and GERD,[2–4] with multiple factors probably contributing to the mechanism. Experts have theorized that a high-fat diet may lead to the prevalence of GERD in the obese,[5] but sufficient data are lacking to make a correlation.

Increased intra-abdominal pressure, lower esophageal sphincter relaxation, and disruption of the esophagogastric junction (hiatal hernia) have all been linked to obesity and probably contribute to the prevalence of GERD.[6] Esophageal dysmotility was identified in critical illness[7] and motility derangements are prevalent throughout the gastrointestinal tract with obesity and likely also contribute to reflux.[8,9] Increased gastric capacity has been associated with obesity, and volumes greater than 30 mL have been associated with risk for aspiration in anesthesia.[10] These changes in normal physiology place obese patients at a potentially increased risk for aspiration during critical illness. Measures to prevent ventilator-associated pneumonia should be used, such as keeping the head-of-bed elevated at least 45° and the use of subglottic suction devices,[11] and these also may help prevent aspiration. H_2 antagonists and proton pump inhibitors are commonly used in the intensive care unit and have been

Disclosure Statement: The authors have nothing to disclose.
[a] Department of Critical Care Medicine, Geisinger Medical Center, 100 North Academy Avenue, Danville, PA 17822, USA
[b] Departments of General Surgery and Critical Care Medicine, Geisinger Medical Center, Temple University Medical School, 100 North Academy Avenue, Mail Code: 20-37, Danville, PA 17822, USA
* Corresponding author.
E-mail address: mreed@geisinger.edu

Crit Care Clin 26 (2010) 625–627
doi:10.1016/j.ccc.2010.06.006
0749-0704/10/$ – see front matter © 2010 Published by Elsevier Inc.

criticalcare.theclinics.com

shown to reduce gastric pH and decrease secretions,[12] although they may not decrease the risk of a chemical pneumonitis because gastric bile acid can also cause severe inflammation.[10]

Several studies have shown an association between increases in BMI and intra-abdominal hypertension (defined as an intra-abdominal pressure [IAP] >12 mm Hg).[13,14] This baseline increase in IAP can predispose obese individuals to developing abdominal compartment syndrome (ACS). ACS occurs when the intra-abdominal pressure exceeds 20 mm Hg with evidence of organ dysfunction, such as oliguria, decreased cardiac output from impedance on venous return, decreased pulmonary compliance, increased intracranial pressure, and lactic acidosis. Disorders such as ascites, intra-abdominal hemorrhage, visceral edema, bowel distension, or large abdominal tumors can lead to ACS.[15] Treatment is usually focused at the cause (ie, paracentesis for massive ascites) and sometimes may require surgical decompression.

NAFLD is a significant problem in obese patients, being present in nearly 75% of obese persons compared with almost 30% of the general population.[16,17] It has a very strong association with diabetes and the metabolic syndrome, and insulin resistance is thought to contribute to disease progression.[18] NAFLD covers a spectrum of disease, from asymptomatic elevations of alanine transaminase to steatosis with lobular inflammation and ballooning degeneration, termed nonalcoholic steatohepatitis (NASH) to liver fibrosis and cirrhosis.[19] Approximately 3% of people with asymptomatic NAFLD progress to cirrhosis, compared with almost 20% of people with NASH.[20] This is fact important in critical care, because cirrhosis has been linked to mortality in critical illness[21] and early hepatic dysfunction.[22] Some patients diagnosed with NAFLD likely may actually have NASH or cirrhosis, which could lead to complications, particularly prolonged drug metabolism and relative immune suppression of liver disease, and worse outcomes in the intensive care unit.

Cholelithiasis is a common disorder. Obesity is a well-documented risk factor for the development of cholesterol stones. The mechanism behind this is thought to be related to the activity of visceral adipose tissue and the metabolic syndrome. Insulin resistance develops and leads to hyperinsulinemia. Hyperinsulinemia may cause increase hepatic excretion of cholesterol and lead to gallbladder dysmotility, which in turn leads to the right environment for stone formation.[23] Gallstones can be asymptomatic but could lead to disorders that may complicate critical illness, such as cholecystitis, cholangitis, and pancreatitis.

REFERENCES

1. El-Serag H. Role of obesity in GORD-related disorders. Gut 2008;57(3):281–4.
2. Corley DA, Kubo A, Zhao W. Abdominal obesity, ethnicity and gastro-oesophageal reflux symptoms. Gut 2007;56(6):756–62.
3. Nilsson M, Johnsen R, Ye W, et al. Obesity and estrogen as risk factors for gastroesophageal reflux symptoms. JAMA 2003;290(1):66–72.
4. Suter M, Dorta G, Giusti V, et al. Gastro-esophageal reflux and esophageal motility disorders in morbidly obese patients. Obes Surg 2004;14(7):959–66.
5. Castell DO. Obesity and gastro-oesophageal reflux: is there a relationship? Eur J Gastroenterol Hepatol 1996;8(7):625–6.
6. Friedenberg FK, Xanthopoulos M, Foster GD, et al. The association between gastroesophageal reflux disease and obesity. Am J Gastroenterol 2008;103(8): 2111–22.

7. Kolbel CB, Rippel K, Klar H, et al. Esophageal motility disorders in critically ill patients: a 24-hour manometric study. Intensive Care Med 2000;26(10):1421–7.

8. Quigley EM. Critical care dysmotility: abnormal foregut motor function in the ICU/ITU patient. Gut 2005;54(10):1351–2 [discussion: 1384–90].

9. Gallagher TK, Geoghegan JG, Baird AW, et al. Implications of altered gastrointestinal motility in obesity. Obes Surg 2007;17(10):1399–407.

10. Kalinowski CP, Kirsch JR. Strategies for prophylaxis and treatment for aspiration. Best Pract Res Clin Anaesthesiol 2004;18(4):719–37.

11. Muscedere J, Dodek P, Keenan S, et al. Comprehensive evidence-based clinical practice guidelines for ventilator-associated pneumonia: prevention. J Crit Care 2008;23(1):126–37.

12. Andrews AD, Brock-Utne JG, Downing JW. Protection against pulmonary acid aspiration with ranitidine. A new histamine H2-receptor antagonist. Anaesthesia 1982;37(1):22–5.

13. Frezza EE, Shebani KO, Robertson J, et al. Morbid obesity causes chronic increase of intraabdominal pressure. Dig Dis Sci 2007;52(4):1038–41.

14. Lambert DM, Marceau S, Forse RA. Intra-abdominal pressure in the morbidly obese. Obes Surg 2005;15(9):1225–32.

15. Malbrain ML, Cheatham ML, Kirkpatrick A, et al. Results from the International Conference of Experts on Intra-abdominal Hypertension and Abdominal Compartment Syndrome. I. Definitions. Intensive Care Med 2006;32(11): 1722–32.

16. Browning JD, Szczepaniak LS, Dobbins R, et al. Prevalence of hepatic steatosis in an urban population in the United States: impact of ethnicity. Hepatology 2004; 40(6):1387–95.

17. Nugent C, Younossi ZM. Evaluation and management of obesity-related nonalcoholic fatty liver disease. Nat Clin Pract Gastroenterol Hepatol 2007;4(8):432–41.

18. Pillai AA, Rinella ME. Non-alcoholic fatty liver disease: is bariatric surgery the answer? Clin Liver Dis 2009;13(4):689–710.

19. Levin PD, Weissman C. Obesity, metabolic syndrome, and the surgical patient. Med Clin North Am 2009;93(5):1049–63.

20. Rafiq N, Bai C, Fang Y, et al. Long-term follow-up of patients with nonalcoholic fatty liver. Clin Gastroenterol Hepatol 2009;7(2):234–8.

21. Foreman MG, Mannino DM, Moss M. Cirrhosis as a risk factor for sepsis and death: analysis of the National Hospital Discharge Survey. Chest 2003;124(3): 1016–20.

22. Kramer L, Jordan B, Druml W, et al. Incidence and prognosis of early hepatic dysfunction in critically ill patients–a prospective multicenter study. Crit Care Med 2007;35(4):1099–104.

23. Tsai CJ, Leitzmann MF, Willett WC, et al. Macronutrients and insulin resistance in cholesterol gallstone disease. Am J Gastroenterol 2008;103(11):2932–9.

Immunologic Changes in Obesity

Mitchell K. Craft, DO[a], Mary Jane Reed, MD, FCCM, FCCP[b],*

KEYWORDS

• Obesity • Leptin • Adiponectin • Adipocytes • Macrophage

A growing body of literature suggests multifaceted alterations to the immune function in obese patients compared with a lean cohort. Although treatment in the intensive care unit has an associated risk of infectious complications, which, if any, of these immunologic alterations are causal is unclear.[1]

Because of recent recognition of their role in inflammatory and immunologic cascades, adipocytes are no longer considered simply a reservoir of energy. White adipose tissue (WAT) is known to house macrophages, leukocytes, and preadipocytes. Obesity is associated with a denser array of macrophages within the adipose tissue. In lean hosts, macrophages represent approximately 10% of the cellularity, but may approach 40% to 50% in obese patients.[2] Adipose tissue macrophages have been associated with the production and release of several proinflammatory cytokines and chemokines ligands, such as tumor necrosis factor (TNF)-α, interleukin (IL)-6, IL-12, IL-10, IL-1β, RANTES (regulated on activation, normal T-cell expressed and secreted), and MIP (macrophage inflammatory protein)-1.[2–4]

WAT also contains preadipocytes, which promote macrophage activation and differentiation through macrophage colony-stimulating factor and peroxisome proliferation-activated receptor gamma. Likewise, an increase in downstream inflammatory mediators occurs, contributing to the chronic inflammatory state of obesity. Toll-like receptors (TLRs) are an assortment of receptors that are crucial in innate immunity. Adipose and other immune cells express TLRs, and seem to be inducible. Alone and with activation of nuclear factor (NF)-κB, enhanced expression of TNF-α and IL-6 again occurs.[5–9]

Adipocytes produce signaling molecules known as *adipokines*. Leptin and adiponectin are two such molecules that have been associated with immunoregulation. Leptin is vital to both energy homeostasis and modulation of the immune response. T-cell proliferation and antiapototic activities are related to leptin, as is T-cell

The authors have nothing to disclose.

[a] Division of Critical Care Medicine, Geisinger Medical Center, 100 North Academy Avenue, Danville, PA 17822, USA

[b] Departments of General Surgery and Critical Care Medicine, Geisinger Medical Center, Temple University Medical School, 100 North Academy Avenue, Mail Code: 20–37, Danville, PA 17822, USA

* Corresponding author.

E-mail address: mreed@geisinger.edu

activation. Secondarily, leptin increases IL-2, which influences CD8 T-cell proliferation; increases concentration of interferon γ; and inhibits IL-4 production. T-cell function is further modulated by leptin through its amplification of adhesion molecules very late activation antigen 2 (VLA-2) and intracellular adhesion molecular 1 (ICAM-1).[10–12]

Leptin has also been associated with macrophage phagocytic activity, and the increased oxidative burst capacity of monocytes and polymorphonuclear leukocytes.[13–15] In obese patients, leptin has been implicated in the persistent elevation of markers of neutrophil activation, myeloperoxidase and calprotectin.[16] In animal models, obese leptin-deficient mice have increased plasminogen activator inhibitor-1 (PAI-1) levels. Through inhibiting plasminogen, PAI-1 is related to impaired fibrin clearance, with resultant increased thrombosis. Clinically, this is likely to render increased myocardial infarction and venous thrombotic risks.[17]

Adiponectin is also an adipokine that has vast systemic function. In general, adiponectin elicits anti-inflammatory, antidiabetic, insulin sensitizing, and antiatherogenic effects. Obesity is associated with diminished adiponectin concentrations. Adiponectin responds to hyperglycemia or TNF-α at the level of endothelial cells through production of nitric oxide and reduces reactive oxygen species, ameliorating inflammatory effects.[18] In animal models, adiponectin has also shown to inhibit progression of atherosclerotic lesions, respond to and mitigate traumatic vascular injury, and ameliorate hypertension.[19–22] In mice with induced myocardial infarction, adiponectin seems to protect against ischemia-reperfusion injury through suppressing TNF-α, apoptosis, and oxidative stress.[23]

Certainly, additional research is needed in humans; however, obesity clearly causes abundant alterations to the immune system. Overall, the aggregate effect seems to be chronic activation of inflammatory mediators. Critical illness also mediates a profound effect on inflammatory, immunologic, endothelial, and thrombotic pathways. The combined effect must be better delineated, with hopes of developing specific interventions to enhance the care of these complex patients.

REFERENCES

1. Winkelman C, Maloney B. Obese ICU patients: resource utilization and outcomes. Clin Nurs Res 2005;14:303–23.
2. Weisberg SP, McCann D, Desai M, et al. Obesity is associated with macrophage accumulation in adipose tissue. J Clin Invest 2003;112:1796–808.
3. Gordon S, Taylor PR. Monocyte and macrophage heterogeneity. Nat Rev Immunol 2005;5:953–64.
4. Odegaard J, Ricardo-Gonzalez R, Goforth M, et al. Macrophage-specific PPARγ controls alternative activation and improves insulin resistance. Nature 2007;447:1116–20.
5. Tontonoz P, Hu E, Spiegelman BM. Stimulation of adipogenesis in fibroblasts by PPAR γ 2, a lipid-activated transcription factor. Cell 1994;79:1147–56.
6. Karagiannides I, Pothoulakis C. Obesity, innate immunity and gut inflammation. Curr Opin Gastroenterol 2007;23(6):661–6.
7. Vitseva O, Tanriverdi K, Tchkonia T, et al. Inducible toll-like receptor and NF-κB regulatory pathway expression in human adipose tissue. Obesity 2008;16:932–7.
8. Auwerx J. PPARγ: a versatile metabolic regulator. Int J Obes 2000;24:S4.
9. Plotkin B, Paulson D, Chelich A, et al. Immune responsiveness in a rat model for type II diabetes (Zucker rat, fa = fa): susceptibility to Candida albicans infection and leucocyte function. J Med Microbiol 1996;44:277–83.

10. Martin-Romero C, Santos-Alvarez J, Goberna R, et al. Human leptin enhances activation and proliferation of human circulating T lymphocytes. Cell Immunol 2000;199:15.
11. Fantuzzi G, Faggioni R. Leptin in the regulation of immunity, inflammation and hematopoiesis. J Leukoc Biol 2000;68:437–46.
12. Falagas M, Kompoti M. Obesity and infection. Lancet Infect Dis 2006;6:438–46.
13. Arsenijevic D, Onuma H, Pecqueur C, et al. Disruption of the uncoupling protein-2 gene in mice reveals a role in immunity and reactive oxygen species production. Nat Genet 2000;26:435–9.
14. Lord G, Matarese G, Howard J, et al. Leptin modulates the T-cell immune response and reverses starvation-induced immunosuppression. Nature 1998; 394:897.
15. Nijhuis J, Rensen S, Slaats Y, et al. Neutrophil activation in morbid obesity, chronic activation of acute inflammation. Obesity 2009;17(11):2014–8.
16. Loskutoff DJ, Samad F. The adipocytes and hemostatic balance in obesity: studies of PAI-1. Arterioscler Thromb Vasc Biol 1998;18:1–6.
17. Goldstein B, Scalia RG, Ma X. Protective vascular and myocardial effects of adiponectin. Nat Clin Pract Cardiovasc Med 2009;6(1):27–35.
18. Okamoto Y, Kihara S, Ouchi N, et al. Adiponectin reduces atherosclerosis in apolipoprotein E-deficient mice. Circulation 2002;106:2767–70.
19. Ohashi K, Kihari S, Ouchi N, et al. Adiponectin replenishment ameliorates obesity-related hypertension. Hypertension 2006;47:1108–16.
20. Okamoto Y, Arita Y, Nishida M, et al. An adipocyte-derived plasma protein, adiponectin, adheres to injured vascular walls. Horm Metab Res 2000;32:47–50.
21. Tao L, Gao E, Jiao X, et al. Adiponectin cardioprotection after myocardial ischemia/reperfusion involves the reduction of oxidative/nitrative stress. Circulation 2007;115:1408–16.
22. Shibata R, Sato K, Pimentel D, et al. Adiponectin protects against myocardial ischemia-reperfusion injury through AMP kinase- and COX-2-dependent mechanisms. Nat Med 2005;11:1096–103.
23. Jay D, Hitomi H, Griendling K, et al. Oxidative stress and diabetic cardiovascular complications. Free Radic Biol Med 2006;40:183–92.

Endocrine System and Obesity

Doyle D. Ashburn, DO[a], Mary Jane Reed, MD, FCCM, FCCP[b],*

KEYWORDS

- Endocrine • Obesity • Diabetes mellitus • Adipokines • Leptin

Obesity is associated with significant alterations in endocrine function. An association with type 2 diabetes mellitus and dyslipidemia has been well documented, typically in conjunction with an obesity-induced metabolic syndrome.[1] The mechanism is likely due to the systemic affects of adipose tissue via the actions of adipokines.[2] Lipoprotein metabolism has implications in inflammation and sepsis, and thyroid dysfunction has been studied as well, indicating a possible connection between body mass index (BMI) and thyroid function.[3,4] Lastly, a rare disorder involving dysfunction of the urea cycle has been identified in patients after gastric bypass surgery.[5] The critical care provider needs to keep these changes in mind when managing the obese patient.

Hyperglycemia first was described by Claude Bernard in 1878 in a patient with hemorrhagic shock, and it is now a well recognized problem in critical illness.[6] Obesity is a well known risk factor for type 2 diabetes and glucose intolerance.[1] The detrimental effects of hyperglycemia in critical illness include increased mortality, incidence of infection, critical illness polyneuropathy, renal insufficiency, transfusion requirement, and increases in ventilator days and intensive care unit (ICU)/hospital length of stay. Intensive insulin therapy may be of benefit, but it is a source of considerable debate.[7] Present blood glucose goals are variable based on investigators. The current recommendation from the Surviving Sepsis Guidelines[8] is a goal blood glucose level under 150 mg/dL. Despite the lack of a consensus in the literature, obese patients should be monitored closely for hyperglycemia, and insulin therapy should be used to control glucose variability.

The increased incidence of hyperglycemia in the obese population is likely a result of acute insulin resistance that is similar to the metabolic syndrome, a condition seen in obesity that takes years to develop.[6] This disorder is characterized by increased insulin resistance, hypertension, obesity (predominantly abdominal), and dyslipidemia. These patients have a higher incidence of coronary artery disease, stroke, peripheral vascular disease, and type 2 diabetes mellitus, thus increasing their medical

[a] Department of Critical Care Medicine, Geisinger Medical Center, 100 North Academy Avenue, Danville, PA 17822, USA
[b] Departments of General Surgery and Critical Care Medicine, Geisinger Medical Center, Temple University Medical School, 100 North Academy Avenue, Mail Code: 20–37, Danville, PA 17822, USA
* Corresponding author.
E-mail address: mreed@geisinger.edu

Crit Care Clin 26 (2010) 633–636
doi:10.1016/j.ccc.2010.06.002
0749-0704/10/$ – see front matter © 2010 Published by Elsevier Inc.

criticalcare.theclinics.com

comorbidities complicating critical illness. Additionally there has been a link to increased cardiovascular events and mortality rates.[1] These patients also develop a proinflammatory and prothrombotic state, leading to an increased risk for venous thromboembolic events.[9,10]

The metabolic syndrome is most likely caused by the synthetic function of the adipose tissue itself. The effects of increased adipose mass have been studied extensively in recent years, and it has been realized that adipose is not just a passive storage site for excess energy, but that it is a multifunctional organ with significant paracrine and endocrine activity via cytokines or chemokines, collectively termed adipokines. The result is usually a proinflammatory state due to elevations of these secretory factors, leading to endothelial damage and promoting atherosclerosis.[2] Increases in adipose tissue have been associated with elevations of inflammatory mediators such as interleukin (IL)-6, IL-8, and tumor necrosis factor (TNF)-α, as well as angiotensin II, which is linked to hypertension and possibly promotes adipokine expression. These increases additionally have been associated with elevations in plasminogen activator inhibiter-1, which is linked to thrombosis and insulin resistance.[2] Adiponectin, another adipokine, has potent vasculoprotective, anti-inflammatory, and antiatherogenic properties and may play a role in glucose management. Obesity leads to decreased levels of adiponectin, promoting atherogenesis and insulin resistance.[1] Adiponectin levels have been shown to be reduced in critical illness, and they may play a role in the development of hyperglycemia.[6,11] Despite these obvious negative effects of adipose tissue, obesity seems to have a paradoxic effect on mortality in critical illness,[12] and it has been proposed that there is an immune-modulating effect of certain adipokines.[13–15] The adipokine leptin is an important mediator of appetite, and it has been shown to be elevated in obesity.[2] Leptin also has been found to have significant immunologic effects, and increased levels were noted in survivors of sepsis.[13] Future research into the endocrine function of adipose tissue could lead to more reliable biomarkers of sepsis, novel metabolic therapies, and possibly change the way the management of obese patients in the ICU is approached.

Hypercholesterolemia is more likely to be seen in obese subjects when compared with the nonobese.[16] In the long term, this has been associated with an increase in atherosclerosis and cardiovascular events, but in acute critical illness, this may have a survival benefit. In fact, low levels of high-density lipoprotein (HDL) have been associated with worse outcomes in severe sepsis.[17] The immune-modulating effects of HDL have been well documented, and HDL may play a role in binding endotoxins, attenuation of adhesion molecule expression, endothelial nitric oxide synthase activation, and antioxidant function, ultimately providing a benefit in disorders where systemic inflammation plays a pivotal role.[18] This population of patients is more likely to be on statin therapy for dyslipidemia. Recent interest in the anti-inflammatory properties of the statins has led to investigation into their role in sepsis. Retrospective studies have suggested a benefit of statins with systemic infections,[19] but a recent prospective cohort showed no difference in outcome.[20] Despite this, it seems reasonable to continue pre-existing statin therapy in absence of any contraindications.

Changes in BMI and levels of thyroid-stimulating hormone have been linked in multiple reports, suggesting a possible link between obesity and hypothyroidism,[3,4,21] while others have shown no relationship.[22] Given that hypothyroidism may be associated with failure to wean from mechanical ventilation,[23] monitoring for evidence of hypothyroidism is warranted in the critically ill obese patient.

Fenves and colleagues[5] reported five cases of fatal hyperammonemic encephalopathy after gastric bypass surgery. Hu and colleagues[24] had reported a similar case that was felt to be related to an ornithine transcarbamylase (OTC) deficiency, possibly due to a genetic mutation. OTC is an important enzyme in the urea cycle, the essential pathway for the disposal of ammonia, and its deficiency is the most common urea cycle disorder. Fenves and colleagues[5] noted no such genetic alterations but felt that a combination of down-regulation of urea cycle enzymes by hyperinsulinemia (caused by gastric bypass surgery) and inhibition of OTC function by zinc deficiency led to elevated ammonia levels and encephalopathy. This is a rare complication of bariatric surgery, but it is important to be aware of this for early recognition.

REFERENCES

1. Levin PD, Weissman C. Obesity, metabolic syndrome, and the surgical patient. Med Clin North Am 2009;93(5):1049–63.
2. Hauner H. Secretory factors from human adipose tissue and their functional role. Proc Nutr Soc 2005;64(2):163–9.
3. Fox CS, Pencina MJ, D'Agostino RB, et al. Relations of thyroid function to body weight: cross-sectional and longitudinal observations in a community-based sample. Arch Intern Med 2008;168(6):587–92.
4. Knudsen N, Laurberg P, Rasmussen LB, et al. Small differences in thyroid function may be important for body mass index and the occurrence of obesity in the population. J Clin Endocrinol Metab 2005;90(7):4019–24.
5. Fenves A, Boland CR, Lepe R, et al. Fatal hyperammonemic encephalopathy after gastric bypass surgery. Am J Med 2008;121(1):e1–2.
6. Jernas M, Olsson B, Sjoholm K, et al. Changes in adipose tissue gene expression and plasma levels of adipokines and acute-phase proteins in patients with critical illness. Metabolism 2009;58(1):102–8.
7. Fahy BG, Sheehy AM, Coursin DB. Glucose control in the intensive care unit. Crit Care Med 2009;37(5):1769–76.
8. Dellinger RP, Levy MM, Carlet JM, et al. Surviving Sepsis Campaign: international guidelines for management of severe sepsis and septic shock: 2008. Crit Care Med 2008;36(1):296–327.
9. Gendall KA, Raniga S, Kennedy R, et al. The impact of obesity on outcome after major colorectal surgery. Dis Colon Rectum 2007;50(12):2223–37.
10. Mullen JT, Davenport DL, Hutter MM, et al. Impact of body mass index on peri-operative outcomes in patients undergoing major intra-abdominal cancer surgery. Ann Surg Oncol 2008;15(8):2164–72.
11. Venkatesh B, Hickman I, Nisbet J, et al. Changes in serum adiponectin concentrations in critical illness: a preliminary investigation. Crit Care 2009;13(4):R105.
12. O'Brien JM Jr, Phillips GS, Ali NA, et al. Body mass index is independently associated with hospital mortality in mechanically ventilated adults with acute lung injury. Crit Care Med 2006;34(3):738–44.
13. Bornstein SR, Licinio J, Tauchnitz R, et al. Plasma leptin levels are increased in survivors of acute sepsis: associated loss of diurnal rhythm, in cortisol and leptin secretion. J Clin Endocrinol Metab 1998;83(1):280–3.
14. Druml W. ICU patients: fatter is better? Intensive Care Med 2008;34(11):1961–3.
15. Marik PE. The paradoxical effect of obesity on outcome in critically ill patients. Crit Care Med 2006;34(4):1251–3.
16. Panagiotakos DB, Pitsavos C, Skoumas Y, et al. Abdominal obesity, blood glucose and apolipoprotein B levels are the best predictors of the incidence of hypercholesterolemia (2001–2006) among healthy adults: the ATTICA study. Lipids Health Dis 2008;7:11.

17. Chien JY, Jerng JS, Yu CJ, et al. Low serum level of high-density lipoprotein cholesterol is a poor prognostic factor for severe sepsis. Crit Care Med 2005; 33(8):1688–93.

18. Murch O, Collin M, Hinds CJ, et al. Lipoproteins in inflammation and sepsis. I. Basic science. Intensive Care Med 2007;33(1):13–24.

19. Tleyjeh IM, Kashour T, Hakim FA, et al. Statins for the prevention and treatment of infections: a systematic review and meta-analysis. Arch Intern Med 2009;169(18): 1658–67.

20. de Saint Martin L, Tandé D, Goetghebeur D, et al. Statin use does not affect the outcome of acute infection: a prospective cohort study. Presse Med 2010;39(3): e52–7.

21. Verma A, Jayaraman M, Kumar HK, et al. Hypothyroidism and obesity. Cause or effect? Saudi Med J 2008;29(8):1135–8.

22. Figueroa B, Velez H, Irizarry-Ramirez M. Association of thyroid-stimulating hormone levels and body mass index in overweight Hispanics in Puerto Rico. Ethn Dis 2008;18:151–4, S2.

23. Datta D, Scalise P. Hypothyroidism and failure to wean in patients receiving prolonged mechanical ventilation at a regional weaning center. Chest 2004; 126(4):1307–12.

24. Hu WT, Kantarci OH, Merritt JL 2nd, et al. Ornithine transcarbamylase deficiency presenting as encephalopathy during adulthood following bariatric surgery. Arch Neurol 2007;64(1):126–8.

Venous Thromboembolic Disease and Hematologic Considerations in Obesity

Mitchell K. Craft, DO[a], Mary Jane Reed, MD, FCCM, FCCP[b],*

KEYWORDS

- Obesity • Pulmonary embolism • PAI-1
- Venous thromboembolism • Adipocytes

Thromboembolic disease remains a major contributor to morbidity and mortality in acute care hospitals. Patients who are critically ill have inherent increased thrombotic risk and it appears obesity does as well. There is a surplus of data regarding the incidence of venous thromboembolic (VTE) disease in hospitals and intensive care units (ICU), with variable results. The incidence of deep vein thrombosis (DVT) and pulmonary embolism (PE) is often underestimated because these entities frequently remain unrecognized. Medical patients have a reported absolute hospital risk for DVT of 10% to 20%, whereas critically ill patients' risk may approach 80%.[1] Studies have shown that despite subcutaneous heparin, 7% to 40% of critically ill patients were identified as having DVT on twice-weekly screening Doppler ultrasonography.[2,3] The incidence of pulmonary embolism in hospitalized patients has been best elucidated in autopsy data in which PE was identified in 10% to 15% of general ward patients and 20% to 25% of ICU patients.[4–6] Several studies have implicated obesity or surrogates, such as waist circumference, as independent risk factors for venous thromboembolic disease. Stein's extensive review of the National Hospital Discharge Survey reported a relative risk (RR) of 2.50 for DVT in obese versus nonobese subjects and a relative risk for PE of 2.21. This was most prominent in subjects younger than 40 years of

---

The authors have nothing to disclose.

[a] Division of Critical Care Medicine, Geisinger Medical Center, 100 North Academy Avenue, Danville, PA 17822, USA

[b] Departments of General Surgery and Critical Care Medicine, Geisinger Medical Center, Temple University Medical School, 100 North Academy Avenue, Mail Code: 20–37, Danville, PA 17822, USA

* Corresponding author.

E-mail address: mreed@geisinger.edu

age with RR of 5.20 and 5.19 for DVT and PE, respectively.[7–10] In addition, there seems to be an incremental risk for recurrent venous thromboembolism with increasing body mass index (BMI).[11] Obesity is related to the metabolic syndrome, which may also independently increase venous thrombotic risks, although there seems to be conflicting data. Astonishingly, there is some data suggestive of improved mortality in cases of acute VTE with increasing body mass index and obesity. Although this analysis controlled many major cofounding risks, it did not directly address patients who are critically ill.[12]

There are several proposed mechanisms for the increased risk for VTE in obese patients. Because of limitations of body habitus, these patients are often less ambulatory and assisted mobilization in the hospital may also be limited. In addition, prophylactic measures may be inadequate. Compression devices are less likely to fit properly, and there is limited data on pharmacologic prophylaxis dosing in the obese. In the ICU, there may well be an increased device-related or procedure-related risk, particularly with central venous catheter placement. Both of these increased procedural complications exist in this patient population, and limited intravenous access may increase duration of central access. Diagnosis may also be compromised. Studies have shown that clinical signs of a DVT are often absent. One study reported a mere 1.5% occurrence of clinical signs.[13] Entities involved in critical illness (resuscitation, sedation, and so forth) and obesity are almost certain to further impair these findings. Furthermore, venous duplex ultrasonography stands to be limited by common critical care entities, such as obesity, edema, dressings, fixators, and so forth.

Obesity has been incriminated in the accelerated pathogenesis of thrombotic conditions, such as myocardial infarction and venous thromboembolism, as early as the 1950s. There has since been a multitude of changes to hemostasis and the delicate balance between thrombus formation and lysis in obesity that have been elucidated. Evolving literature implicates plasminogen activator inhibitor-1 (PAI-1) as a cause of increased thrombosis in obese patients. PAI-1 disrupts the conversion of plasminogen to plasmin, in turn decreasing fibrinolytic activity. Adipocytes produce PAI-1 and further regulation by tumor necrosis factor α and IL-1 is suspected. In both animal and human models, PAI-1 is noted to increase with obesity. As there are increasing levels of PAI-1, tissue plasminogen activator (t-PA) and urokinase-derived plasminogen activation are reduced with consequential impaired fibrin clearance and promotion of thrombus.[14–17] Adiponectin is an adipocytokine linked to several antiatherogenic and antithrombotic mechanisms. Levels of adiponectin are inversely related to BMI, with deficiency being associated with enhanced thrombus formation and platelet aggregation. Obesity is also related to increased levels of von Willebrand factor, which in turn increases platelet aggregation.[18–21] In addition, endothelial tissue-type plasminogen activator (t-PA), a key enzyme in the fibrinolytic response, appears to have a diminished release in obese patients, which is also linked with accelerated thrombogenisis.[22,23] A recent study investigated the prevalence of several known and measurable thrombophilias in subjects preparing for bariatric surgery. In comparison to the prevalence in the general population, these subjects had statistically significant increases in factors VIII, IX, and XI as well as lupus anticoagulant, all of which has an ascribed increased risk for thrombosis.[24]

Venous thromboembolic disease continues to be a major source of morbidity and mortality, with obese patients who are critically ill presenting some of the most at-risk patients. As the literature evolves, it has become clear that there is a complex relationship between obesity and thrombosis and atherogenesis. It is true that many of these conditions are reversible with weight loss; however, obesity remains on the rise. Management of obese patients must incorporate and consider these intricate changes in an attempt to improve patient outcomes.

REFERENCES

1. Geerts W, Bergqvist D, Pineo G, et al. Prevention of venous thromboembolism the seventh ACCP Conference on antithrombotic and thrombolytic therapy. Chest 2006;126(3):338S–400S.
2. Hirsch DR, Ingenito EP, Goldhaber SZ. Prevalence of deep venous thrombosis among patients in medical intensive care. JAMA 1995;274:335–7.
3. Marik PE, Andrews L, Maini B. The incidence of deep venous thrombosis in ICU patients. Chest 1997;111:661–4.
4. Stein P, Henry J. Prevalence of acute pulmonary embolism among patients in a general hospital and at autopsy. Chest 1995;108(4):978–81.
5. Moser KM, LeMoine JR, Nachtwey FJ, et al. Deep venous thrombosis and pulmonary embolism: frequency in a respiratory intensive care unit. JAMA 1981;246: 1422–4.
6. Neuhaus A, Bentz RR, Weg JG. Pulmonary embolism in respiratory failure. Chest 1978;73:460–5.
7. Borch K, Braekkan S, Mathiesen E, et al. Anthropometric measures of obesity and risk of venous thromboembolism. Arterioscler Thromb Vasc Biol 2010;30:121–7.
8. Stein P, Beemath A, Olson R. Obesity as a risk factor in venous thromboembolism. Am J Med 2005;118:978–80.
9. Goldhaber S, Grodstein F, Stampfer M, et al. A prospective study of risk factors for pulmonary embolism in women. JAMA 1997;277(8):642–5.
10. Hansson P, Welin L, Tibblin G, et al. Deep vein thrombosis and pulmonary embolism in the general population "The study of Men born in 1913". Arch Intern Med 1997;157(15):1665–70.
11. Eichenger S, Hron G, Bialonczyk C, et al. Overweight, obesity and the risk of recurrent venous thromboembolism. Arch Intern Med 2008;168(15):1678–83.
12. Barba R, Zapatero A, Losa JE, et al. Body mass index and mortality in patients with acute venous thromboembolism: findings from the RIETE registry. J Thromb Haemost 2008;6(4):595–600.
13. Geerts W, Code K, Jay R, et al. A prospective study of venous thromboembolism after major trauma. N Engl J Med 1994;331:1601–6.
14. Sartori MT, Danesin C, Saggiorato G, et al. The PAI-1 gene 4 G/5 G polymorphism and deep vein thrombosis in patients with inherited thrombophilia. Clin Appl Thromb Hemost 2003;9(4):299–307.
15. Loskutoff D, Samad F. The adipocyte and hemostatic balance in obesity studies of PAI-1. Arterioscler Thromb Vasc Biol 1998;18:1–6.
16. Levi M, Biemond BJ, van Zonneveld AJ, et al. Inhibition of plasminogen activator inhibitor-1 activity results in promotion of endogenous thrombolysis and inhibition of thrombus extension in models of experimental thrombosis. Circulation 1992;85: 305–12.
17. Alessi M, Vague I. PAI-1 and the metabolic syndrome links, causes and consequence. Arterioscler Thromb Vasc Biol 2006;26:2200–7.
18. Kato H, Kashiwagi H, Shiraga M, et al. Adiponectin acts as an endogenous antithrombotic factor. Arterioscler Thromb Vasc Biol 2006;26(1):224–30.
19. Basili S, Pacini G, Guagnano MT, et al. Insulin resistance as a determinant of platelet activation in obese women. J Am Coll Cardiol 2006;48(12):2531–8.

20. Mertens I, Van Gaal LF. Obesity, haemostasis and the fibrinolytic system. Obes Rev 2002;3(2):85–101.
21. Warlow C, McNeill A, Ogston D, et al. Platelet adhesiveness, coagulation and fibrinolytic activity in obesity. J Clin Pathol 1972;25:484–6.
22. Carmeliet P, Schoonjans L, Kieckens L, et al. Physiological consequences of loss of plasminogen activator gene function in mice. Nature 1994;368(6470):419–24.
23. Van Guilder G, Hoetzer G, Smith D, et al. Endothelial t-PA release is impaired in overweight and obese adults but can be improved with regular aerobic exercise. Am J Physiol Endocrinol Metab 2005;289:807–13.
24. Overby DW, Kohn GP, Cahan MA, et al. Prevalence of thrombophilias in patients presenting for bariatric surgery. Obes Surg 2009;19(9):1278–85.

Airway Management in the Obese Patient

William A. Loder, MD[a,b,*]

KEYWORDS

• Intubation • Airway • Laryngoscope • Obese

Any patient can have a difficult airway, but obese patients have anatomic and physiologic features that can make airway management particularly challenging. Changes in respiratory mechanics, such as a decreased functional residual volume, may result in rapid onset of hypoxemia in the obese patient. Excess soft tissue around the neck and in the oropharynx can make mask ventilation difficult or impossible. Increased intra-abdominal pressure from abdominal adiposity increases the risk of regurgitation and aspiration.

To effectively manage airways in obese patients, health care providers working in the intensive care unit (ICU) setting must be proficient in airway evaluation and management in all types of patients. They need to be skilled in mask ventilation and direct laryngoscopy. The providers need to know how to safely manage a difficult airway situation, both anticipated and unanticipated[1–4] and should be familiar with the American Society of Anesthesiology's Difficult Airway Algorithm (**Fig. 1**).

It is unclear whether obese patients are at an increased risk of difficulty associated with endotracheal intubation. Studies focusing on obesity as a risk factor for airway problems have reported a wide range of risks. One study found that obese individuals (body mass index [BMI]>35, calculated as the weight in kilograms divided by the height in meters squared) were 7 times more likely to have a difficult intubation,[5] but in a study of more than 90,000 intubations, obesity was shown to be a statistically significant but weak predictor of difficult intubation, with an odds ratio of only 1.34.[6] In a study using the intubation difficulty scale (IDS),[7] 105 obese patients were compared with 99 nonobese patients. The obese patients had higher average IDS scores, but all the patients were intubated successfully using direct laryngoscopy. The average time to intubation was 46 seconds in the obese group. The lowest oxygen saturation reported for any patient was 97%.[8] Another study found no relationship between BMI, neck circumference, or obstructive sleep apnea and difficult intubations.[9]

The author has no financial or other conflicts of interest to disclose.
[a] Department of Anesthesiology, Geisinger Medical Center, Danville, PA 17822-2025, USA
[b] Department of Critical Care Medicine, Geisinger Medical Center, Danville, PA 17822-2025, USA
* Department of Anesthesiology, Geisinger Medical Center, Danville, PA 17822-2025.
E-mail address: wloder@geisinger.edu

Crit Care Clin 26 (2010) 641–646
doi:10.1016/j.ccc.2010.08.002
0749-0704/10/$ – see front matter © 2010 Elsevier Inc. All rights reserved.
criticalcare.theclinics.com

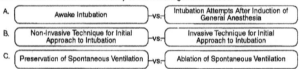

DIFFICULT AIRWAY ALGORITHM

1. Assess the likelihood and clinical impact of basic management problems:
   A. Difficult Ventilation
   B. Difficult Intubation
   C. Difficulty with Patient Cooperation or Consent
   D. Difficult Tracheostomy

2. Actively pursue opportunities to deliver supplemental oxygen throughout the process of difficult airway management

3. Consider the relative merits and feasibility of basic management choices:

   A. Awake Intubation —vs— Intubation Attempts After Induction of General Anesthesia

   B. Non-Invasive Technique for Initial Approach to Intubation —vs— Invasive Technique for Initial Approach to Intubation

   C. Preservation of Spontaneous Ventilation —vs— Ablation of Spontaneous Ventilation

4. Develop primary and alternative strategies:

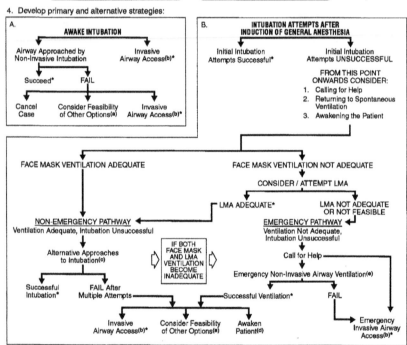

* Confirm ventilation, tracheal intubation, or LMA placement with exhaled CO_2

a. Other options include (but are not limited to): surgery utilizing face mask or LMA anesthesia, local anesthesia infiltration or regional nerve blockade. Pursuit of these options usually implies that mask ventilation will not be problematic. Therefore, these options may be of limited value if this step in the algorithm has been reached via the Emergency Pathway.

b. Invasive airway access includes surgical or percutaneous tracheostomy or cricothyrotomy.

c. Alternative non-invasive approaches to difficult intubation include (but are not limited to): use of different laryngoscope blades, LMA as an intubation conduit (with or without fiberoptic guidance), fiberoptic intubation, intubating stylet or tube changer, light wand, retrograde intubation, and blind oral or nasal intubation.

d. Consider re-preparation of the patient for awake intubation or canceling surgery.

e. Options for emergency non-invasive airway ventilation include (but are not limited to): rigid bronchoscope, esophageal-tracheal combitube ventilation, or transtracheal jet ventilation.

Fig. 1. Difficult Airway Algorithm. LMA, laryngeal mask airway. (*From* American Society of Anesthesiologists Task Force on Management of the Difficult Airway. Practice guidelines for management of the difficult airway: an updated report by the American Society of Anesthesiologists Task Force on Management of the Difficult Airway. Anesthesiology 2003;98:1273; with permission.)

There have been several studies on multiple risk factors including the Mallampati score, thyromental distance, cervical spine extension, interincisor distance, upper lip bite test,[10,11] neck circumference, and BMI. Three articles[11–13] have calculated the positive and negative predictive values (PPV and NPV, respectively) of several of these individual risk factors. None of the factors have a PPV greater than 50% but all have an NPV greater than 95%.

Several studies have examined a combination of factors, trying to improve on the prediction of a difficult airway. One study[12] on the combination of neck circumference (>43 cm) and Mallampati score (>3) found that the combination was better than either factor alone with a PPV of 44%. Another article[14] on the combination of the Mallampati score (>3) and thyromental distance (<6 cm) demonstrated improved prediction of difficult intubation. Rao and colleagues[15] reported that positioning obese patients so that the ear is aligned with the sternal notch (the ramp position) seemed to facilitate tracheal intubation. Another article on the combination of a class III upper lip bite test (unable to bite upper lip with lower incisors) with the interincisor, thyromental, or sternomental distances reported that all 3 combinations had low PPVs.[16] All this confirms the clinical impression that the prediction of difficult intubation is, at best, imprecise.[14,17,18] If a patient tests positive for any risk factor, there may be a difficulty in intubation and obesity is one additional factor to be taken into consideration. The more risks that individuals have the more likely they are to have a difficult airway and intubation. If individuals test negative for all risk factors, they are unlikely to have a difficult airway and intubation.

In addition to the aforementioned risk factors that suggest a difficult airway, there are additional factors that must be considered when managing a patient's airway. Clinical conditions such as a cervical spine injury, full stomach, and intravascular volume status influence the management of the airway. In addition, patients in the ICU who require endotracheal intubation are frequently hypoxic, hypercapnic, and/ or hypotensive, which add to the complexity and the urgency of the situation. Before any attempt to instrument an airway, it is vital that the patient be, at least briefly, evaluated. Essential equipment should be gathered. The exact list of equipment needed may vary slightly depending on the intubating individual's preference, but endotracheal tubes with stylets, functioning suction, a bag-valve device connected to an oxygen source, laryngoscope and blades, oral/nasal airways, and a device to detect end-tidal carbon dioxide are essential.

Nonemergent potentially difficult airways should be managed conservatively. Additional help and equipment should be sought, and a plan to safely intubate the patient should be formulated. There are many ways of handling the anticipated difficult airway and they depend on the individual's training, the techniques that the individual is comfortable with, and the patient's condition. The possibilities include, but are not limited to, maintaining bag ventilation until help arrives, placing a supraglottic airway device, performing an awake intubation with a flexible fiberoptic bronchoscope, or proceeding with direct laryngoscopy. The best method depends on the skills and experience of the individuals involved.

In the ICU setting, evaluation of the airway can be difficult, and if initial intubation attempts fail, the situation can quickly deteriorate and become life threatening. Between 8% and 12% of intubations in the ICU are difficult, usually defined as 2 or more attempts by someone skilled in direct laryngoscopy.[19–21] In the unanticipated difficult intubation, the skills and knowledge of the individual managing the airway are of paramount importance if a disaster is to be avoided. Obese patients are especially difficult to manage. When compared with nonobese patients, obese patients desaturate more rapidly and recover from hypoxia more slowly. In obese patients, effective bag-mask ventilation may be very difficult or impossible and they are at an increased risk for aspiration.[13,22] An increased neck size can make retrograde wire intubation and emergent surgical airway procedures difficult. To add to the complexity, many of the techniques used to manage difficult airways are a bit toilsome in the obese patient. The effective use of adjunctive devices, such as flexible broncho-scopes, supraglottic devices, and lightwands,[23,24] requires the acquisition and prac-tice of a specific set of skills that a given intensivist may or may not have. As described earlier, health care providers who deal with airways must have the abilities to safely manage them and must know when to ask for help. In case of a failed intubation, consideration should be given to calling for help early before the situation becomes irretrievable with a catastrophic patient outcome.

There is controversy regarding whether hypnotics or neuromuscular blocking agents should be given to facilitate intubation. Some individuals prefer to support and assist a patient's respiratory efforts and intubate a patient with spontaneous respiration. Others think that having a patient asleep and paralyzed improves mask ventilation and laryngoscopy and makes intubation easier. Both methods have advan-tages and disadvantages. Giving a muscle relaxant may make laryngoscopy easier and decrease the chances of difficult intubation,[25] but if the patient is paralyzed and cannot be intubated, the airway has to be maintained until the intubation can be successfully accomplished or the patient returns to spontaneous respiration. In obese patients, maintaining an adequate airway, particularly after multiple intubation attempts, can be challenging. Like so many other areas of medicine, clinical judgment and a low threshold to ask for additional expertise are required.

In review, there is little difference in how the airway is approached in obese and nonobese patients. Obesity does not seem to be an independent risk factor for difficult intubation but is one of the several factors that need to be considered as part of an airway evaluation. However, if an obese patient cannot be intubated, maintaining an adequate airway is more likely to be challenging and may lead to a "cannot intubate, cannot ventilate" situation. Patients in the ICU are frequently unstable and need to be intubated in a relatively emergent manner. This sense of urgency can lead to mistakes, with the occasional disastrous outcome. Health care providers who manage airways and intubate patients need to have the skills, experience, and confidence to do so safely.

In summary, the risk of a difficult airway/intubation situation in an obese patient is similar to that in the nonobese patient. In addition, individuals who manage airways and endotracheally intubate patients as part of their practice need to be skilled at bag-mask ventilation and direct laryngoscopy. Some individuals prefer using a short or stubby laryngoscope handle when dealing with obese patients. These individuals should also be proficient with at least 1 alternative method of airway management, such as flexible fiberoptic bronchoscope, supraglottic devices (LMA, COBRA PLA, EngineeredMedical Systems, IN, USA), lightwand, or video laryngoscopy. There are several types of rigid stylets as well as more invasive techniques, such as transtra-cheal jet ventilation, retrograde wire techniques, and emergent cricothyrotomy. Finally, knowing how to quickly evaluate an airway and when to call for help, either before or after the difficulty is encountered, are critical skills and judgments that must be acquired by anyone dealing with the airway.

REFERENCES

1. Langeron O, Amour J, Vivien B, et al. Clinical review: management of difficult airways. Crit Care 2006;10:243–7.
2. Rose DK, Cohen MM. The airway: problems and predictions in 18,500 patients. Can J Anaesth 1994;41:372–83.
3. Walz JM, Zayaruzny M, Heard SO. Airway management in critical illness. Chest 2007;131:608–20.

4. Drolet P. Management of anticipated difficult airway—a systematic approach: continuing professional development. Can J Anaesth 2009;56:683–701.
5. Juvin P, Lavaut E, Dupont H, et al. Difficult tracheal intubation is more common in obese than in lean patients. Anesth Analg 2003;97:595–600.
6. Lundstrom LF, Moller AM, Rosenstock C, et al. High body mass index is a weak predictor for difficult and failed tracheal intubation. Anesthesiology 2009;110: 266–74.
7. Adnet F, Borron SW, Racine SX, et al. The intubation difficulty scale (IDS): proposal and evaluation of a new score characterizing the complexity of endotracheal intubation. Anesthesiology 1997;87:1290–7.
8. Lavi R, Segal D, Ziser A. Predicting difficult airways using the intubation difficulty scale: a study comparing obese and non-obese patients. J Clin Anesth 2009;21: 264–7.
9. Neligan PJ, Porter S, Max B, et al. Obstructive sleep apnea is not a risk factor for difficult intubation in morbidly obese patients. Anesth Analg 2009;109:1182–6.
10. Salimi A, Farzanegan B, Rastegarpour A, et al. Comparison of the upper bite test with measurement of thyromental distance for prediction of difficult intubations. Acta Anaesthesiol Taiwan 2008;46(2):61–5.
11. Eberhart L, Arndt C, Cierpka T, et al. The reliability and validity of the upper lip bite test compared with the Mallampati classification to predict difficult laryngoscopy an external prospective evaluation. Anesth Analg 2005;101(1):284–9.
12. Gonzalez H, Minville V, Delanoue K, et al. The importance of increased neck circumference to intubation difficulties in obese patients. Anesth Analg 2008;106:1132–6.
13. Kheterpal S, Han R, Tremper KK, et al. Incidence and predictors of difficult and impossible mask ventilation. Anesthesiology 2006;105:885–91.
14. Shiga T, Wajima Z, Inoue T, et al. Predicting difficult intubation in apparently normal patients. Anesthesiology 2005;103:429–37.
15. Rao SL, Kunselman AR, Schuler HG, et al. Laryngoscopy and tracheal intubation in the head elevated position in obese patients: a randomized, controlled equivalence trial. Anesth Analg 2008;107:1912–8.
16. Khan ZH, Mohammadi M, Rasouli MR, et al. The diagnostic value of the upper lip bite test combined with sternomental distance, thyromental distance and interincisor distance of prediction of easy laryngoscopy and intubation: a prospective study. Anesth Analg 2009;109:822–4.
17. Karkouti K, Rose DK, Wigglesworth D, et al. Predicting difficult intubation: a multivariable analysis. Can J Anaesth 2000;47:730–9.
18. Lee A, Fan LT, Gin T, et al. A systematic review (meta-analysis) of accuracy of the Mallampati test to predict the difficult airway. Anesth Analg 2006;102:1867–78.
19. Schwartz DE, Matthay MA, Cohen NH. Death and other complications of emergency airway management in critically ill adults. A prospective investigation of 297 tracheal intubations. Anesthesiology 1995;82:367–76.
20. Jaber S, Amraoui J, Lefrant JY, et al. Clinical practice and risk factors for immediate complications of endotracheal intubation in the intensive care unit: a prospective, multiple-center study. Crit Care Med 2006;34:2355–61.
21. Griesdale DE, Bosma TL, Kurth T, et al. Complications of endotracheal intubation in the critically ill. Intensive Care Med 2008;34:1835–42.
22. Yildiz TS, Solak M, Toker K. The incidence and risk factors of difficult mask ventilation. J Anesth 2005;19:7–11.
23. Wong SY, Coskunfirat ND, Hee HI, et al. Factors influencing time of intubation with a lightwand device in patients without known airway abnormality. J Clin Anesth 2003;16:326–31.

24. Dhonneur G, Abdi W, Ndoko SK, et al. Video-assisted versus conventional tracheal intubation in morbidly obese patients. Obes Surg 2009;19:1096–101.
25. Lundstrom LH, Moller AM, Rosenstock C, et al. Avoidance of neuromuscular blocking agents may increase the risk of difficult tracheal intubation: a cohort study of 103812 consecutive adult patients recorded in the Danish Anaesthesia Database. Br J Anaesth 2009;103:283–90.

Vascular Procedures in the Critically Ill Obese Patient

Omar Rahman, MD[a,b,*], Laurel Willis, PA-C[b]

KEYWORDS

- Obese • Body mass index • Central venous catheter
- Procedure • Ultrasonography • Critically ill

The increasing societal prevalence of obesity is consequential to the increasing number of critically ill obese patients. A large number of bariatric procedures have also resulted in a growing exposure of intensivists to this population. Up to 26% of patients in the intensive care unit (ICU) may be obese, and the prevalence of morbid obesity or superobesity is likely to increase as well.[1–4] (In this article, patients with body mass index [BMI] 35–50 kg/m^2 and BMI >50 kg/m^2, calculated as the weight in kilograms divided by the height in meters squared, are referred to as morbidly severely obese and superobese patients, respectively.)

Bedside vascular procedures are an essential aspect of care in critically ill patients. An estimated 5 million central venous catheters (CVCs) are placed yearly in the United States.[5] In ICUs, establishing vascular access, administration of central-acting medications, and hemodynamic monitoring are some of the well-established indications of central venous and arterial cannulation (**Boxes 1** and **2**).

Although aspects of pathophysiology, pharmacokinetics, and general care of critically ill obese patients have been reviewed, not many trials or descriptions of vascular procedures are available in this population. Generally, these procedures are deemed challenging, especially in the severely obese and superobese groups.[2,4]

This article reviews the general, anatomic and physiologic considerations pertaining to vascular procedures in critically ill obese patients. In addition, the use of ultrasonography (USG) for these procedures is discussed.

[a] Adult Intensive Care/Shock Trauma Unit, Geisinger Medical Center, Danville, PA, USA
[b] Department of Critical Care Medicine, Geisinger Medical Center, MC 20-37, 100 North Academy Avenue, Danville, PA 17822, USA
* Corresponding author. Department of Critical Care Medicine, Geisinger Medical Center, MC 20-37, 100 North Academy Avenue, Danville, PA 17822.
E-mail address: orahman2@geisinger.edu

Crit Care Clin 26 (2010) 647–660
doi:10.1016/j.ccc.2010.08.003
0749-0704/10/$ – see front matter © 2010 Elsevier Inc. All rights reserved.

criticalcare.theclinics.com

Box 1
Common bedside vascular procedures in the critically ill patient

Peripheral intravenous catheter

CVCs

    Sites

        Subclavian, internal jugular, femoral veins

    Types

        Traditional single, double, triple, quadrangle, or 5-lumen catheters (7F to 8.5F)

        Single lumen introducer catheter (8.5F to 10.5F or 14 to 16 gauge)

        Hemodialysis catheter

        CVC for endovascular hypothermia

Pulmonary artery catheters

Arterial catheters

    Sites

        Radial, femoral, axillary, brachial

    Types

        3F to 5F

        18 to 20 gauge

ANATOMIC CONSIDERATIONS

Vascular procedures in the obese have been described as high risk primarily because of anatomic concerns[2,4] Ambiguity in identifying anatomic landmarks for vascular procedures in critically ill obese patients is a function not only of their body habitus but also of the state of their underlying acute illness. Volume depletion, airway compromise, severe hypoxemic respiratory failure, coagulopathy, edematous states, ecchymosed extremities, and fractured limbs are some of the conditions that further exacerbate that anatomic conundrum.

Head and Neck Region

The sternal notch, margins of the sternocleidomastoid muscle, and contour of the clavicle help identify the course of the vascular bundles in the head and neck in non-obese patients. These, among other, surface landmarks traditionally described for jugular (internal and external) and subclavian venous cannulation may be obscured in severely morbidly obese patients. Large neck circumference, short neck height, skinfolds, and excess adipose tissue in the neck and chest wall are factors that contribute to anatomic complexity. Lack of palpable identification of the trachea, thyroid cartilage, carotid pulsation, and borders of the clavicle are commonly encountered by the operator while assessing for neck access in a morbidly obese patient. Moreover, the descriptions of variable anatomic relation between internal jugular vein (IJV) and carotid artery as well between the right and left IJV demonstrated by ultrasonography only further compounds the issue.[6–8]

Inguinal Region and Extremities

Femoral vascular access is confronted by similar problems. In a severely obese patient, palpation of the iliac crest, anterior superior iliac spine, pubic symphysis,

---

Box 2
Common indications for vascular procedures in the critically ill patient

Intravenous (IV) access

    Inability to establish peripheral venous access

    Hemodynamic instability requiring central venous access

    Massive transfusion and/or active resuscitation

Medications requiring central infusion

    Vasoactive agents

    Hypertonic solutions

Total parenteral nutrition

Hemodynamic monitoring

    Arterial pressure monitoring

    Mixed or central venous oxygen saturation

    Cardiac output and other pulmonary artery catheter variables measurement

Therapeutic hypothermia

Renal replacement therapy (intermittent or continuous)

Plasmapheresis

Chemotherapy

Extended-term IV access

    Prolonged antibiotics

    Miscellaneous

---

and pulsations of the femoral artery is not possible at times. The identification of the femoral triangle as well as the traditional VAN mnemonic (medial to lateral: vein, artery, nerve) may not be applicable because the procedure is frequently attempted much lower from the inguinal ligament in the presence of excess adipose tissue and multiple skinfolds. Moreover, the effects of an abdominal pannus overlying the inguinal areas prohibit access to the femoral triangle and also pose impediment to smooth procedural operation and infection control measures.

Peripheral venous access may be similarly impaired in the upper limbs, especially in the setting of earlier described coexisting conditions, particularly in edematous states. Antecubital veins and veins in the arm are less likely to be accessible compared with forearm veins. Arterial access, in particular, is challenging because palpation of radial, brachial, and axillary pulses may be markedly cumbersome in obese patients. Axillary arterial cannulation using the pectoralis muscles and the clavicle as landmarks cannot be performed in the presence of large amounts of axillary adiposity and folds.

Peripheral venous access is virtually impossible in the legs and feet of severely obese patients with critical illness. The presence of chronic dependent edema is an additional inhibiting factor.

GENERAL PROCEDURAL CONSIDERATIONS
Location of the Procedure

Most vascular access procedures in critically ill patients are done in ICUs, emergency departments (EDs), or by anesthesia personnel in operating rooms. The size of the room, resource availability, and urgency of the procedure impact the ease or difficulty of performing that procedure. In most ICUs and EDs, room space may be compromised by the presence of an oversized bariatric bed or mattress for the obese patient. The size of the room obviously varies. As an example, in 3 different ICUs in the authors' institution, the room sizes are 14 × 12, 12 × 12, and 20 × 14 ft. It is clear that a smaller-sized ICU or an ED room with an oversized bed can seriously limit room for maneuverability during preparation and performance of such procedures.

During an initial resuscitation process, there may be several infusion pumps, a mechanical ventilator, multiple tubing, supply cabinet, and care team personnel in the room while preparing for a vascular procedure. Unless procedures are being done in a cardiac arrest or near-arrest situation in which sterility is not of primary concern, the operators may face difficulty in preparing a sterile table and maintaining a sterile field for the procedure.

Even when active resuscitation is not an issue, the exercise may be challenging in limited space, especially when arterial catheters or pulmonary artery catheters (PACs) are being placed, which require connecting hemodynamic pressure tubing, or while using ultrasound (US) during the procedure.

Availability of specific bariatric ICU rooms may be a useful concept; however, this concept is likely to be an uncommon scenario because of resource use, high patient turnover in large institutions, and triage concerns.

Patient Positioning

Trendelenburg position is the preferred position for CVC placement above the diaphragm to achieve higher central venous volume and larger vein caliber and to prevent air embolism. In the morbidly severely obese and superobese critically ill patients, positioning as such may be problematic. Reduced lung volumes, diminished pulmonary reserve, effects of intra-abdominal pressure (IAP), elevated right heart pressures, and difficult airway-related issues can potentially lead to marked acute deterioration of cardiopulmonary status in this population. Caution must be undertaken while performing these procedures in mechanically ventilated unstable obese patients with hypoxemia and shock states. It may be prudent to use the Trendelenburg position only after complete sterile field preparation, topical anesthetic instillation, and operator preparation.

Central Line "Bundles"

Maintenance of the sterile technique during insertion is the major determinant of catheter-related infection and bacteremia. The development of bundles and processes of care have positively impacted catheter-related infection rates. Educational method and insertion checklists have shown to significantly reduce these infections and other associated risks of insertion.[9,10] However, in morbidly obese patients, there are some important practical considerations:

1. Subclavian site: Most infection control guidelines and recommendations suggest that the subclavian site should be the preferred site of a CVC placement because of its lower risk of infection.[11–13] In severely obese patients, attempts at subclavian insertion without identifiable anatomic landmarks may be high risk. This condition is particularly true for patients who have high FiO_2 or positive end-expiratory pressure requirements. A pneumothorax or hemothorax may be life threatening because of its hemodynamic effects and also because detection (clinical or radiological) of these conditions in morbidly obese patients may be missed or delayed. Ultrasonography and color flow Doppler methods may be used in such circumstances,

although subclavian access via this method is less studied and more limited compared with internal jugular or femoral venous US-guided insertion.[14]

2. Antiseptic solution application: Chlorhexidine gluconate (CHG) is the preferred skin antiseptic solution for percutaneous vascular insertions, although povidone-iodine can be used in some circumstances.[15,16] These solutions are available in the form of CHG sponge brushes (cholrapreps, CareFusion, El Paso, TX, USA), wipes, sponges, or liquid solutions. In the femoral or neck regions, the presence of multiple skinfolds and adipose tissue may require careful and innovative application of this solution to ensure adequate antisepsis. Preparation for solution application in obese patients may include neck position modification as well as relocating thick skinfolds and/or pannus from the insertion site by using ties, tape, or restraints. Careful application of solution is even more important in situations in which an indwelling catheter is being exchanged over guidewire in obese patients.

3. Maximal barrier precautions: For patients with large body surface area, more than one large sterile body drape may be required. Moreover, the drapes should be positioned keeping in mind the anatomic intricacies of the chosen site.

4. Daily assessment of line necessity: Removal of unnecessary intravascular devices is a major prevention against infection. Morbidly obese critically ill patients are at risk of having catheters longer than needed because of their difficult access status and procedural risks.[2,4] In these patients, the necessity for temporary catheters must be assessed in a manner similar to that in nonobese patients. Peripherally inserted central catheters (PICCs) or tunneled catheter placement early in the course of critical illness may be required to avoid this complication.[17]

Catheter Insertion Technique

A modified version of the technique described by Seldinger[19] and Aubaniac[18] is currently used to insert vascular catheters over a guidewire. Cannulation of the vessel percutaneously by a hollow bore needle is followed by advancement of a guidewire into the vessel. Several steps of the insertion process may need modification in the morbidly obese population:

1. Local anesthesia: Because of the presence of excess skin folds and subcutaneous tissue, the volume of intradermal and subcutaneous infiltration with 1% lidocaine must be judicious and the administration must be directed by US guidance.

2. The depth and angle of needle insertion using either surface landmarks or US guidance differ greatly in obese patients. In one study using US guidance, jugular vein depth and diameter in bariatric patients with an average BMI of 49 kg/m^2 was 15 ± 4.3 mm and 16 ± 6.4 mm, respectively.[20]

3. Tissue dilation: Small scalpel skin incision followed by insertion of a dilator over the wire is required to open the skin and dilate the subcutaneous track with rotational movement for smooth insertion of the venous catheter. In obese patients, this step has the potential for misdirected dilation due to excess irregular adipose tissue. If the angle of the dilator insertion varies greatly from the initial angle of needle insertion, forming an irregular track and resultant bending or distortion of the guidewire is possible. In some instances, the distortion of the wire may not allow the catheter to be inserted smoothly and may also raise the danger of unraveling or breaking of the guidewire when it is finally removed after the catheter has been inserted.

4. Length and position: The tip of the CVC should ideally be in the distal superior vena cava (SVC). Peres[21] described a formula based on patient's height to determine the final length of neck CVCs. The formula has been shown to correlate with the position of the catheter tip at the atriocaval junction.[22] As studies dispute the accuracy

of traditional height-based formulas,[23] guidewires should preferentially be inserted 2 cm beyond the final determined length of the catheter or in most cases, 18 cm should be considered the upper limit of safe guidewire introduction.[24] Because specific formulas based on BMI are lacking, a meticulous consideration of catheter length is required in obese patients based on body surface area, vessel depth, and anatomy.

5. Securing arterial and venous catheters with skin sutures may require extra care in obese patients, especially in the case of catheters in the head and neck. Presence of a short neck or skinfold may require careful positioning of the external portion of a 16-, 20-, or 30-cm catheter.

6. Portable chest radiographs in severely obese and superobese patients with excess soft tissue shadow or overlying breast tissue can hinder radiographic determination of the catheter tip. Intra-atrial US guidance was used in such patients successfully to confirm catheter placement and to evaluate for pneumothorax.[20]

US-GUIDED CATHETER INSERTION
General Principles

Two-dimensional ([2-D]; B-mode) USG is mostly used for vascular catheterization. Higher-frequency probes (7.5–15 MHz) are usually used for US-guided catheter insertion; however, lower-frequency (5 MHz) probes may be used in severely obese patients to access deep vessels.[25] Blood vessels are hypoechoic, appearing dark in contrast to isoechoic, gray soft tissue. Differentiation between artery and vein is essential. Arteries are pulsatile, except in severe hypotension or cardiac arrest. Veins are generally compressible in the absence of luminal thrombus or other obstruction. In the upper extremities, small arteries, such as radial and brachial arteries, may be seen as compressible vessels. Color flow and pulsed wave Doppler imaging can define nature of vascular flow.

USG Catheter Insertion: CVC

USG vascular device insertion was first advocated in 1984.[26] Despite several decades of successful use of surface landmarks to insert central catheters, the notion of reduction of insertion-related complications and improved ease of insertion using USG was exciting. Over the last 2 decades, several small studies demonstrated the efficacy of US-guided catheter insertion over landmark methods in jugular, femoral, and, to a lesser extent, subclavian venous catheter insertions.[27–32] The meta-analysis by Randolph and colleagues[14] in 1996 of 8 randomized trials involving 513 catheter placements estimated that real-time USG for CVC insertion is associated with a significant reduction in placement failures (relative risk [RR], 0.32; 95% confidence interval CI, 0.18–0.55), decreased insertion complications (RR, 0.22; 95% CI, 0.10–0.45), and reduced number of venipunctures during attempts (RR, 0.60; 95% CI, 0.45–0.79). Another meta-analysis in 2003 by Hind and colleagues[33] of 18 trials with 1646 participants estimated that 2D US-guided catheter insertion for IJV cannulation in adults was associated with a significantly lower overall (RR, 0.14; 95% CI, 0.06–0.33) and first-attempt (RR, 0.59; 95% CI, 0.39–0.88) failure rates. Limited data also favored femoral and subclavian venous USG catheter insertion in adults in that analysis. In a larger study by Karakitsos and colleagues[34] in which US-guided internal jugular insertion was successful 100% of the time compared with 94% in the landmark method (900 patients; 450 each group, $P<.001$), morbidly obese patients were not included.

Obesity has been identified as a risk factor for surface landmark–guided CVC placement,[2,4,20,25,35] but controlled studies are limited. In 1998, a report of 30 of 32 successful IJV US-guided catheter insertions included 8 patients with no visual or palpable landmarks, but details specific to that group were not listed.[36] Fujiki and colleagues[37] compared simulated IJV puncture using US guidance in nonobese patients (BMI <30 kg/m^2) to morbidly obese patients (BMI >40 kg/m^2). Although no difference in success rates was observed between the 2 groups, US-guided catheter insertion was recommended for morbidly obese patients because of increased observed overlap of the IJV and carotid artery in that group. Brusasco and colleagues[20] studied the safety and efficacy of USG catheter insertion in 55 severely obese patients (BMI 49 $\pm$ 7 kg/m^2) undergoing bariatric surgery. US-guided was used for vein cannulation and also performed after guidewire insertion to demonstrate the guidewire's presence in the SVC or right atrium (RA) before catheter placement. Successful catheterization was shown in all cases without complications, such as arterial puncture, hematoma, or pneumothorax. Concordance was seen between chest radiograph and ultrasonic findings with intra-atrial electrocardiogram.

CVC insertion training incorporating real-time US-guided techniques may provide additional valuable learning benefits for new operators. This knowledge may improve the success rate of insertion of CVCs without US guidance. Simulation training has demonstrated improved identification of the desired veins with US guidance compared with landmark techniques.[38]

US-Guided Catheter Insertion: Other Catheter Types

In addition to CVC placement, US guidance has been used with demonstrated success in other circumstances, such as arterial cannulation and peripheral intravenous (PIV) catheter insertion.

Trials of US-guided arterial catheter placement for radial artery cannulation compared with those of palpation method have demonstrated success.[39–41] Case studies for successful insertion of brachial and axillary artery catheters are reported.[42,43] Studies specific to arterial catheters in obese patients are lacking.

Successful use of USG for PIV has been well described.[44–49] Studies have evaluated US-guided PIV insertion in the emergency room.[44–46,49] One study by Brannam and colleagues[44] reported successful use of USG to place PIV by nurses in the emergency room after a simulation course in difficult-access cases. Of the 321 patients studied, 28% were obese. Keyes and colleagues[46] published a study demonstrating successful US-guided cannulation of basilic and brachial veins in difficult access patients using a 7.5 MHz probe. Of the 100 patients studied, 21 were obese, and a 91% success rate was demonstrated. In contrast, a recent work by Stein and colleagues[49] showed no difference in success rates for PIV insertion in US-guided versus non-US-guided catheter placement. In this randomized trial of 59 patients (28 US-guided and 31 non-US-guided), the number of overweight patients was much higher in the group (36% vs 12%) in which USG was used. Moreover BMI and vessel characteristics (depth, caliber) were not described.

PICC insertion is gaining widespread acceptance and may be an acceptable substitute for CVCs for certain indications (eg, long-term intravenous access or parenteral nutrition).[17] US guidance has also been demonstrated to improve the insertion of PICCs.[50,51]

Because US guidance in real time for CVC insertion (with or without Doppler) reduces the number of venipuncture attempts, increases insertion success rate, and reduces complications associated with catheter placement in the general critically ill population, it is more likely to be of benefit in a high-risk catheter insertion situation such as obesity. The authors recommend the use of US guidance for arterial catheter placement and CVC placement, especially in severely obese patients in the ICU.

SPECIAL CONSIDERATIONS
Hemodynamic Monitoring

Common hemodynamic monitoring variables in patients in the ICU include arterial blood pressure (ABP), central venous pressure (CVP), central or pulmonary venous oxygen saturation, cardiac output (CO), stroke volume (SV), and relative indices (cardiac index, SV index [SVI]). The pathophysiologic cardiovascular and respiratory changes ascribed to obesity may impact the measurement of these variables.

ABP

An accurate blood pressure (BP) measurement in the critically ill patient is essential for guiding therapy. Continuous ABP measurement via an invasive arterial catheter is frequently required in patients in the ICU. In the severely obese patient, the need for ABP monitoring is related to the use of ABP values as a hemodynamic measurement tool and also necessitated at times because of the inaccurate nature of traditional cuff measurements of BP in this population. Normally, to obtain the most accurate BP measurement, the cuff bladder should be greater than or equal to 80% of the patient's arm circumference, and the width of the cuff should be greater than or equal to 40% of the arm circumference. In the critical obese patient, especially with shock states, cuff measurements may be inadequate. In such patients, if BP cuffs are placed on the patient's wrist, ankles, legs, or thighs, the readings are potentially erroneous and may misguide the clinician. Arterial catheter placement may be the preferred means of ABP monitoring in such patients. Accuracy of ABP can be of concern sometimes in the severely obese patient because of the presence of increased atherosclerosis, arterial wall thickness, and overlying tissue thickness.

PAC placement and measurement of CO, SV, and related indices

PAC insertion in the morbidly obese can be challenging because of the duration of the procedure and complications of inserting a relatively short-length large bore introducer mounted on a dilator.[52] In addition, interpretation of obtained hemodynamic indices based on BMI in critically ill patients is considered uncertain, especially at extremes of ranges. Severe obesity may be associated with increase in CO, RA pressure, right ventricular end diastolic pressure, and pulmonary artery mean and occlusive pressures.[53–55] In obese patients, fat-free body mass is a strong correlate of SV and CO.[54] Elevated CVP can be seen because of increased intrathoracic pressure associated with a higher IAP in the severely obese or abdominal surgical procedures involving pneumoperitoneum.[56–58]

In a retrospective study by Stelfox and colleagues,[59] the relationship of BMI to CO and SV was assessed in 700 patients who underwent cardiac catheterization and were found to have disease-free coronary arteries. Each 1 kg/m^2 increase in BMI was associated with an increase of 0.08 L/min (95% CI, 0.06–0.10; P = .001) in CO and an increase of 1.35 mL (95% CI, 0.96–1.74; P = .001) in SV. No BMI association was seen with cardiac index (0.003 $L/min/m^2$; 95% CI, 0.008–0.014; P = .571) or the SVI (0.17 mL/m^2; 95% CI, 0.03– 0.37; P = .094). A similar relationship between BMI and both CO and SV was noted when patients were classified into BMI categories. The investigators concluded that body surface area indexing to CO and SV attenuate the effect of BMI. Mechanical ventilation details, presence of shock, and severity of illness were not described fully in the studied population.

Other semi-invasive vascular hemodynamic tools

Pulse contour analysis uses peripheral arterial pressure waveforms to continuously calculate CO and estimate SV. Various calibration- and noncalibration-based tools are available. Pulmonary thermodilution (PiCCO, PULSION Medical Systems, Munich, Germany) and lithium indicator dilution (LiDCO Ltd, Lake Villa, IL, USA) are calibrated techniques, whereas FloTrac using Vigileo monitors is a noncalibrated method for the calculation of CO, SV, and stroke volume variation (SVV). These newer methods have been validated in studies; however, the data for the accuracy and reliability of these methods in morbidly obese critically ill patients are currently limited.[60–65] SVV may be a useful guide to assess fluid responsiveness in the morbidly obese patient.[66] A study by Mayer and colleagues[67] on 15 obese (BMI>30 kg/m^2) versus 23 nonobese patients undergoing coronary artery bypass grafting demonstrated adequate agreement of CO and cardiac index by FloTrac/Vigileo (Edwards Lifesciences Corp, Irvine, CA, USA) analysis compared with bolus pulmonary artery thermodilution in both groups.

Therapeutic Hypothermia

Application of mild hypothermia to prevent anoxic brain injury after ventricular fibrillation (V-Fib) cardiac arrest is an accepted standard of care.[68–70] Hypothermia or sustaining normothermia is used in other settings as well, including non–V-Fib cardiac arrests and intracranial hypertension management among others.[71–73] Both surface cooling and endovascular methods are used to achieve target temperature. Because goals of therapy are to achieve rapid cooling of body temperature, controlled maintenance at desired temperature, and accurate rate of rewarming, it is apparent that surface cooling devices may be of limited utility in severely obese and superobese patients because of larger body surface area.

Endovascular cooling methods include different commercial products that involve central venous placement of a cooling catheter. Catheters such as the Alsius CoolGard 3000/Icy (ZOLL Medical Corporation, Chelmsford, MA, USA) or the Accutrol/Innercool (Philips Healthcare Andover, MA, USA) system can be placed in the femoral vein so that core body cooling is achieved by temperature modulation in the inferior vena cava. Other catheter types are also available. In patients with a BMI greater than 30 kg/m^2, endovascular cooling may be superior to surface methods.[74] In the morbidly obese patient population, therapeutic hypothermia should be preferably attempted using intravascular methods.

Intraosseous Access

Intraosseous (IO) access has been used effectively in emergent access situations for pediatric patients.[75,76] The role of IO access has expanded to involve adult trauma and inpatients.[77–79] In patients with otherwise difficult peripheral access because of dehydration, limb injury, or shock, cannulation of the intramedullary venous plexus may be lifesaving. Leidel and colleagues[79] prospectively studied 10 emergency room patients undergoing resuscitation using both IO and CVC access. The first-attempt success rate for IO insertion was 90% versus 60% for CVC placement. In addition, the mean procedure time was shorter with IO access (2.3 min $\pm$ 0.8 vs 9.9 min $\pm$ 3.7; $P<.001$). BMI or weight characteristics of subjects were not described.

Because tibial or humeral insertions are the most common sites for IO access, it is evident that the use of this strategy is fraught by potential problems in morbidly obese patients. Although IO cannula sets specific to obese patients (eg, EZ-IO LD [Vidacare Corporation, Shavano Park, TX, USA]) are marketed, the data on IO access in obese adults is limited. Newer IO access adults systems involving sternal infusion[80,81] may also be of limited utility in the morbidly obese because of chest wall thickness.

SUMMARY

Obese patients present a unique challenge for vascular access in the ICU population. In this population of patients, such procedures must always be considered high risk, requiring expert operator or supervisor presence. Catheter placement conditions and derivation of data from these devices must always be analyzed in the relevant anatomic or physiologic context. Proper planning, modifiable techniques tailored to the individual patient, and the use of USG are highly recommended, if not essential, elements of safe catheter insertions in these patients.

REFERENCES

1. Ray DE, Matchett SC, Baker K, et al. The effect of body mass index on patient outcomes in a medical ICU. Chest 2005;127(5):2125–31.
2. El-Solh A, Sikka P, Bozkanat E, et al. Morbid obesity in the medical ICU. Chest 2001;120(6):1989–97.
3. Tremblay A, Bandi V. Impact of body mass index on outcomes following critical care. Chest 2003;123(4):1202–7.
4. Pieracci FM, Barie PS, Pomp A. Critical care of the bariatric patient. Crit Care Med 2006;34(6):1796–804.
5. Frasca D, Dahyot-Feizlier C, Mimoz O. Prevention of central venous catheter related infection in the intensive care unit. Crit Care 2010;14:212.
6. Caridi JG, Hawkins IF, Wiechmann BN, et al. Sonographic guidance when using the right internal jugular vein for central vein access. AJR Am J Roentgenol 1998; 171(5):259–63.
7. Turba UC, Flacker R, Hannegan C, et al. Anatomic relationship of the internal jugular vein and the common carotid artery applied to percutaneous transjugular procedures. Cardiovasc Intervent Radiol 2005;28(3):303–6.
8. Samy Modeliar S, Sevestre MA, de Cagny B, et al. Ultrasound evaluation of central veins in the intensive care unit: effects of dynamic maneuvers. Intensive Care Med 2008;34(2):333–8.
9. Berenholtz SM, Pronovost PJ, Lipsett PA, et al. Eliminating catheter-related blood-stream infections in the intensive care unit. Crit Care Med 2004;32(10):2014–20.
10. Warren DK, Zack JE, Mayfield JL, et al. The effect of an education program on the incidence of central venous catheter-associated bloodstream infection in a medical ICU. Chest 2004;126(5):1612–8.
11. Merrer J, De Jonghe B, Golliot F, et al. Complications of femoral and subclavian venous catheterization in critically ill patients: a randomized controlled trial. JAMA 2001;286(6):700–7.
12. Ruesch S, Walder B, Tramèr MR. Complications of central venous catheters: internal jugular versus subclavian access – a systematic review. Crit Care Med 2002;30(2):454–60.
13. Parienti JJ, Thirion M, Mégarbane B, et al. Femoral vs. jugular venous catheteri-zation and risk of nosocomial events in adults requiring acute renal replacement therapy: a randomized controlled trial. JAMA 2008;99(20):2413–22.
14. Randolph AD, Cook DJ, GonzalesCA, et al. Ultrasound guidance for placement of central venous catheters: a meta-analysis of the literature. Crit Care Med 1996;24(12):2053–8.
15. Maki DG, Ringer M, Alvarado CJ. Prospective randomized trial of povidone-iodine, alcohol, and chlorhexidine for prevention of infection associated with central venous and arterial catheters. Lancet 1991;338(8763):339–43.

16. Mimoz O, Pieroni L, Lawrence C, et al. Prospective randomized trial of two anti-septic solutions for prevention of central venous or arterial colonization and infection in intensive care unit patients. Crit Care Med 1996;24(11):1818–23.
17. Al Raiy B, Fakih MG, Bryan-Nomides N, et al. Peripherally inserted central venous catheters in the acute care setting: a safe alternative to high-risk short-term central venous catheters. Am J Infect Control 2010;38(2):149–53.
18. Aubaniac R. L'injection intraveneuse sousclaviculare advantage et technique. Presse Med 1952;60(68):1456.
19. Seldinger SI. Catheter replacement of the needle in percutaneous arteriography: a new technique. Acta Radiol 1953;39(5):368–76.
20. Brusasco C, Corradi F, Zattoni PL, et al. Ultrasound-guided central venous cannulation in bariatric patients. Obes Surg 2009;19(10):1365–70.
21. Peres PW. Positioning central venous catheters-A prospective survey. Anaesth Intensive Care 1990;18(4):536–9.
22. Czepizak CA, O'Callaghan JM. Evaluation of formulas for optimal positioning of central venous catheters. Chest 1995;107(6):1662–4.
23. Joshi AM, Bhosale GP, Parikh GP, et al. Optimal positioning of right-sided internal jugular venous catheters: comparison of intra-atrial electrocardiography versus Peres' formula. Indian J Crit Care Med 2008;12(1):10–4.
24. Andrews RT, Bova DA, Venbrux AC. How much guidewire is too much? Direct measurement of the distance from subclavian and internal jugular vein access sites to the superior vena cava-atrial junction during central venous catheter placement. Crit Care Med 2000;28(1):138–42.
25. Maecken T, Grau T. Ultrasound imaging in vascular access. Crit Care Med 2007; 35(5 Suppl):S178–85.
26. Legler D, Nugent M. Doppler localization of the internal jugular vein facilitates central venous cannulation. Anesthesiology 1984;60(5):481–2.
27. Mallory DL, Shawker TH. Ultrasound guidance improves the success rate of internal jugular vein cannulation. Chest 1990;98(1):157–60.
28. Teichgraber UK, Benter T, Gebel M, et al. A sonographically guided technique for central venous access. AJR Am J Roentgenol 1997;169(3):731–3.
29. Denys BG, Reddy PS. Ultrasound-assisted cannulation of the internal jugular vein. Circulation 1993;87(5):1557–62.
30. Leung J, Duffy M, Finckh A. Real-time ultrasonographically-guided internal jugular vein catheterization in the emergency department increases success rates and reduces complications: a randomized, prospective study. Ann Emerg Med 2006;48(5):540–7.
31. Lefrant JY, Cuvillon P, Benezet JF, et al. Pulsed Doppler ultrasonography guidance for catheterization of the subclavian vein: a randomized study. Anesthesiology 1998;88(5):1195–201.
32. Bold RJ, Winchester DJ, MadaryAR, et al. Prospective randomized trial of Doppler-assisted subclavian vein catheterization. Arch Surg 1998;133:1089–93.
33. Hind D, Calvert N, McWilliams R, et al. Ultrasonic locating devices for central venous cannulation: meta-analysis. BMJ 2003;327(7411):361.
34. Karakitsos D, Labropoulos N, De Groot E, et al. Real-time ultrasound-guided catheterization of the internal jugular vein: a prospective comparison with the landmark technique in critical care patients. Crit Care 2006;10(6):R162.
35. Graham AS, Ozment C, Tegtmeyer K, et al. Central venous catheterization. N Engl J Med 2007;356:e21.
36. Hrics P, Wilber S, Blanda MP, et al. Ultrasound-assisted internal jugular vein catheterization in the ED. Am J Emerg Med 1998;16(4):401–3.

37. Fujiki M, Guta CG, Lemmens HJ, et al. Is it more difficult to cannulate the right internal jugular vein in morbidly obese patients than in non-obese patents? Obes Surg 2008;18(9):1157–9.

38. Barsuk JH, McGaghie WC, Cohen ER, et al. Simulation-based mastery learning reduces complications during central venous catheter insertion in a medical intensive care unit. Crit Care Med 2009;37(10):2697–701.

39. Levin PD, Sheinin O, Gozal Y. Use of ultrasound guidance in the insertion of radial artery catheters. Crit Care Med 2003;31(2):481–4.

40. Sandhu NS, Patel B. Use of ultrasonography as a rescue technique for failed radial artery cannulation. J Clin Anesth 2006;18(2):138–41.

41. Schwemmer U, Arzet HA, Trautner H, et al. Ultrasound-guided arterial cannulation in infants improves success rate. Eur J Anaesthesiol 2006;23(6):476–80.

42. Sandhu NS. The use of ultrasound for axillary artery catheterization through pectoral muscles: a new anterior approach. Anesth Analg 2004;99(2):562–5.

43. Tsao SL, Chen KY, Hsu WT, et al. A modified technique for ultrasound-guided cannulation of radial and brachial arteries in patients with circulation collapse. Acta Anaesthesiol Taiwan 2008;46(2):91–4.

44. Brannam L, Blaivas M, Lyon M, et al. Emergency nurses' utilization of ultrasound guidance for placement of peripheral intravenous lines in difficult-access patients. Acad Emerg Med 2004;11(12):1361–3.

45. Costantino TG, Parikh AK, Satz WA, et al. Ultrasonography-guided peripheral intravenous access versus traditional approaches in patients with difficult intravenous access. Ann Emerg Med 2005;46(5):456–61.

46. Keyes LE, Frazee BW, Snoey ER, et al. Ultrasound-guided brachial and basilic vein cannulation in emergency department patients with difficult intravenous access. Ann Emerg Med 1999;34(6):711–4.

47. Blaivas M, Brannam L, Fernandez E. Short-axis vs long-axis approaches for teaching ultrasound-guided vascular access on a new inanimate model. Acad Emerg Med 2003;10:1307–11.

48. Sandhu NPS, Sidhu DS. Mid-arm approach to basilic and cephalic vein cannulation using ultrasound guidance. Br J Anaesth 2004;93:292–4.

49. Stein JC, Cole W, Kramer N, et al. Ultrasound-guided peripheral intravenous cannulation in emergency department patients with difficult IV access. Acad Emerg Med 2004;11:581–2.

50. Mills CN, Leibmann O, Stone MB, et al. Ultrasonographically guided insertion of a 15cm catheter into the deep brachial or basilic veins in patients with difficult intravenous access. Ann Emerg Med 2007;50(1):68–72.

51. Robinson MK, Mogensen KM, Grudinskas GF, et al. Improved care and reduced costs for patients requiring peripherally inserted central catheters: the role of bedside ultrasound and a dedicated team. JPEN J Parenter Enteral Nutr 2005; 29(5):374–9.

52. Thompson EC, Wilkins HE. Insufficient length of pulmonary artery introducer in an obese patient. Arch Surg 2004;139(7):794–6.

53. Snyder D. Evaluation of the obese patient. In: Longnecker D, Tinker J, Morgan G, editors. Principles and practices of anesthesiology. St Louis (MO): Mosby; 1998. p. 507–27.

54. Collis T, Devereux RB, Roman MJ, et al. Relations of stroke volume and cardiac output to body composition: the strong heart study. Circulation 2001;103(6): 820–5.

55. Pascual M, Pascual DA, Soria F, et al. Effects of isolated obesity on systolic and diastolic left ventricular function. Heart 2003;89(10):1152–6.

56. Lambert DM, Marceau S, Forse RA. Intra-abdominal pressure in the morbidly obese. Obes Surg 2005;15(9):1225–32.
57. El-Dawlatly AA, Al-Dohayan A, Favretti F, et al. Anesthesia for morbidly obese patients: a study of hemodynamic changes during bariatric surgery. Middle East J Anesthesiol 2002;16(4):411–7.
58. Dumont L, Mattys M, Mardirosoff C, et al. Hemodynamic changes during laparoscopic gastroplasty in morbidly obese patients. Obes Surg 1997;7(4):326–31.
59. Stelfox HT, Ahmed SB, Ribeiro RA, et al. Hemodynamic monitoring in obese patients: the impact of body mass index on cardiac output and stroke volume. Crit Care Med 2006;34(4):1243–6.
60. Shoemaker WC, Belzberg H, Wo CC, et al. Multicenter study of noninvasive monitoring systems as alternatives to invasive monitoring of acutely ill emergency patients. Chest 1998;114(6):1643–52.
61. Pittman J, Bar-Yosef S, SumPing J, et al. Continuous cardiac output monitoring with pulse contour analysis: a comparison with lithium indicator dilution cardiac output measurement. Crit Care Med 2005;33(9):2015–21.
62. Bein B, Worthmann F, Tonner PH, et al. Comparison of esophageal Doppler, pulse contour analysis, and real-time pulmonary artery thermodilution for the continuous measurement of cardiac output. J Cardiothorac Vasc Anesth 2004;18(2):185–9.
63. Brumfield AM, Andrew ME. Digital pulse contour analysis: investigating age-dependent indices of arterial compliance. Physiol Meas 2005;26(5):599–608.
64. Horswell J, Worley T. Continuous cardiac output measured by arterial pulse pressure analysis in surgical patients. Crit Care Med 2005;33(12 Suppl):A67.
65. Manecke GR, Peterson M, Auger WR. Cardiac output determination using the arterial pulse wave: a comparison of a novel algorithm against continuous and intermittent thermodilution. Crit Care Med 2004;32(12 Suppl):A43.
66. Jain AK, Dutta A. Stroke volume variation as a guide to fluid administration in morbidly obese patients undergoing laparoscopic bariatric surgery. Obes Surg 2010;20(6):709–15.
67. Mayer J, Boldt J, Beschmann R, et al. Uncalibrated arterial pressure waveform analysis for less-invasive cardiac output determination in obese patients undergoing cardiac surgery. Br J Anaesth 2009;103(2):185–90.
68. Bernard SA, Morley PT, Hoek TL, et al. Treatment of comatose survivors from out-of hospital cardiac arrest with induced hypothermia. N Engl J Med 2002;346(8):557–63.
69. The Hypothermia after Cardiac Arrest Study Group. Mild hypothermia to improve the neurological outcome after cardiac arrest. N Engl J Med 2002;346(8):549–56.
70. Nolan JP, Morley PT, Hoek TL, et al. Advancement Life Support Task Force of the International Liaison Committee on Resuscitation: therapeutic hypothermia after cardiac arrest: an advisory statement by the Advancement Life Support Task Force of the International Liaison committee on Resuscitation. Resuscitation 2003;57(3):231–5.
71. Bernard S. Hypothermia after cardiac arrest: expanding the therapeutic scope. Crit Care Med 2009;37(7 Suppl):S227–33.
72. Polderman KH. Application of therapeutic hypothermia in the intensive care unit. Opportunities and pitfalls of a promising treatment modality—Part 2: practical aspects and side effects. Intensive Care Med 2004;30(5):757–69.
73. Krieger DW, De Georgia MA, Abou-Chebl A, et al. Cooling for acute ischemic brain damage (COOL AID): an open pilot study of induced hypothermia in acute ischemic stroke. Stroke 2001;32(8):1847–54.

74. Steinberg GK, Ogilvy CS, Shuer LM, et al. Comparison of endovascular and surface cooling during unruptured cerebral aneurysm repair. Neurosurgery 2004;55(2):307–14.

75. Rosetti VA, Thompson BM, Miller J, et al. Intraosseous infusion: an alternative route of pediatric intravascular access. Ann Emerg Med 1985;14(9):885–8.

76. American Heart Association in collaboration with the International Liaison Committee on Resuscitation, guidelines for cardiopulmonary resuscitation and emergency cardiovascular care: pediatric advanced life support. Circulation 2005;112(24 Suppl):IV1–203.

77. Brenner T, Bernhard M, Helm M, et al. Comparison of two intraosseous infusion systems for adult emergency medical use. Resuscitation 2008;78(3):314–9.

78. Leidel BA, Kirchhoff C, Braunstein V, et al. Comparison of two intraosseous access devices in adult patients under resuscitation in the emergency department: a prospective, randomized study. Resuscitation 2010;81(8):994–9.

79. Leidel BA, Kirchhoff C, Bogner V, et al. Is the intraosseous access route fast and efficacious compared to conventional central venous catheterization in adult patients under resuscitation in the emergency department? A prospective observational pilot study. Patient Saf Surg 2009;3(1):24.

80. Macnab A, Christenson J, Findlay J, et al. A new system for sternal intraosseous infusion in adults. Prehosp Emerg Care 2000;4(2):173–7.

81. Frascone R, Kaye K, Dries D, et al. successful placement of an adult sternal intraosseous line through burned skin. J Burn Care Rehabil 2003;24(5):306–8.

Ultrasound-Assisted Lumbar Puncture in Obese Patients

Robert Strony, DO

KEYWORDS

- Ultrasound • Lumbar puncture • Obese
- Emergency department

LUMBAR PUNCTURE IN THE OBESE PATIENT

The use of ultrasound to mark landmarks for diagnostic lumbar puncture (LP) has been described in the emergency medicine (EM) and the anesthesia literature.[1–3] Most of the anesthesia literature pertains to elective obstetric patients requiring epidural anesthesia and involves depth and angle calculations.[1,4] One of the most difficult scenarios arises when obese patients (body mass index [BMI] >30) present to an acute care setting, such as the emergency department (ED) or intensive care unit (ICU) and require diagnostic LP. Stiffler and colleagues[3] suggested that the efficiency of ultrasound was inversely related to BMI in identifying bone landmarks for LP. Despite this drawback, the investigators were able to identify landmarks in 75% of obese patients undergoing ultrasound-guided LP in the ED.[3] Ferre and Sweeney[5] concluded that an increased BMI made it more difficult to palpate landmarks but did not affect the ability of ultrasound to identify relevant landmarks; 46% of patients in their study had a BMI greater than 30.[6] In a later study, they reported a 92% success rate using ultrasound-guided landmarks, regardless of BMI.[7]

There has been only 1 randomized controlled trial demonstrating ultrasound-guided LP versus traditional LP in the emergency setting.[8] This study involved patients requiring diagnostic LP who presented to the ED. Patients were randomized to ultrasound-marked landmarks versus palpation of landmarks. The ultrasound-guided landmark technique was 1.32 times more likely to be successful than the traditional palpation landmark technique.[8] In a subgroup analysis of patients with BMI greater than 30, those who underwent ultrasound-guided LP had 100% success (n = 5). This result contrasted to only 4 of the 7 obese patients who had a successful traditional LP. The investigators concluded that ultrasound landmarks were 2.3 times more likely to be successful compared with palpation-guided landmarks in the obese subset.[8]

Department of Emergency Medicine, Geisinger Medical Center, 100 North Academy Avenue, Danville, PA 17822, USA
E-mail address: rjstrony@geisinger.edu

Crit Care Clin 26 (2010) 661–664
doi:10.1016/j.ccc.2010.07.002   **criticalcare.theclinics.com**
0749-0704/10/$ – see front matter © 2010 Elsevier Inc. All rights reserved.

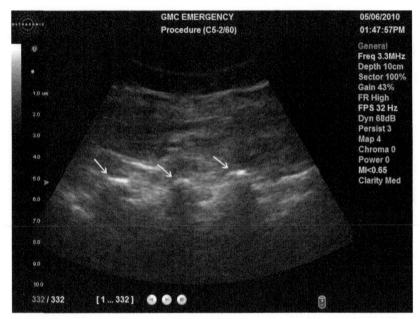

Fig. 1. Sagittal view of lumbar spinous processes L3-L5 using low-frequency 3.3-MHz curvilinear array transducer. The spinous processes are identified as curvilinear hyperechoic bright white lines with black acoustic shadowing posteriorly.

When these patients present to the acute care setting, ultrasound can be an indispensable adjunct to facilitate diagnostic LP in a safe and efficient manner. The method that the ED in the author's medical center uses is similar to the method described by Peterson and Abele[2] and Nonmura and colleagues.[8] The staff consists of board certified EM physicians and EM residents. The patient is positioned in the lateral decubitus or sitting position. A high-frequency 10-MHz linear array transducer is used if the patient has a low BMI, usually less than 30. For a BMI greater than 30 (as shown in the following figures), the low-frequency 3.3-MHz curvilinear probe is used.

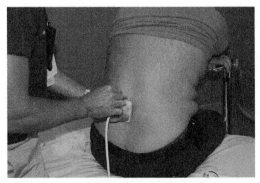

Fig. 2. Patient placed in lateral decubitus position. The midline is identified in the sagittal plane. This patient had a calculated BMI of 35, requiring the use of the low-frequency 3.3-MHz curvilinear array to visualize the spinous processes.

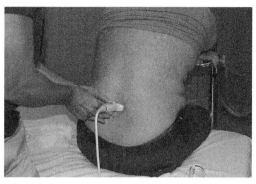

Fig. 3. Transverse probe orientation. A surgical marking pen used to identify the interspinous space by absence of spinous process and acoustic shadowing.

The landmark height is calculated by palpating both superior iliac spines and drawing an imaginary line to connect them. The L3-4 or L4-5 space is identified. The sagittal view is used to establish the midline of spine (delineated by visualizing consecutive spinous processes) (**Fig. 1**). The spinous processes appear as hyperechoic bright curvilinear white lines with posterior shadowing. The probe is placed in the sagittal plane, and marks are made at the superior and inferior aspect of the probe as seen in **Fig. 2**. The dots are then connected with a straight line. The probe is then rotated to the transverse plane as shown in **Fig. 3**. The probe is passed over the spinous processes in the midline until the spinous processes are again identified in

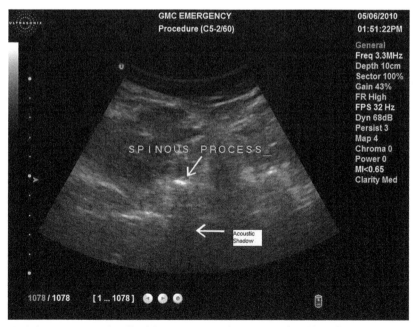

Fig. 4. Spinous process visualized in transverse orientation. After identifying 2 consecutive spinous processes, the interspinous space is identified by the absence of a hyperechoic bright white line and shadowing.

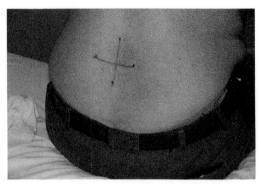

Fig. 5. The intersection of lines made in the sagittal and transverse planes marks the area of needle entry.

the transverse plane (**Fig. 4**). The probe is then moved either superiorly or inferiorly to identify the next spinous process (identified by the hyperechoic line and shadowing artifact) and then the interspinous space, which is identified by an absence of the hyperechoic spinous process and acoustic shadow. A transverse line is then made. The intersection of the sagittal and transverse lines, as shown in **Fig. 5** marks the point of needle entry. Diagnostic LP then proceeds in a standard fashion.

REFERENCES

1. Grau T, Leipold RW, Conradi R, et al. Ultrasound imaging facilitates localization of the epidural space during combined spinal and epidural anesthesia. Reg Anesth Pain Med 2001;26:64–7.
2. Peterson M, Abele J. Bedside ultrasound for difficult lumbar puncture. J Emerg Med 2005;28(2):197–200.
3. Stiffler K, Jwayyed S, Wilber ST, et al. The use of ultrasound to identify pertinent landmarks for lumbar puncture. Am J Emerg Med 2007;25:331–4.
4. Tran D, Kamani AA, Al-Attas E, et al. Single-operator real-time ultrasound-guidance to aim and insert a lumbar epidural needle. Can J Anaesth 2010;57:313–21.
5. Ferre R, Sweeney TW. Emergency physicians can easily obtain ultrasound images of anatomical landmarks relevant to lumbar puncture. Am J Emerg Med 2007;25:291–6.
6. Balki M, Lee Y, Halpern S, et al. Ultrasound imaging of the lumbar spine in the transverse plane: the correlation between estimated and actual depth to the epidural space in obese patients. Anesth Analg 2009;108(6):1876–81.
7. Ferre R, Sweeney TW, Strout TD, et al. Ultrasound identification of landmarks preceding lumbar puncture: a pilot study. Emerg Med J 2009;26:276–7.
8. Nomura J, Leech SJ, Shenbagamurthi S, et al. A randomized control study of ultrasound-assisted lumbar puncture. J Ultrasound Med 2007;26:1341–8.

Bedside and Radiologic Procedures in the Critically Ill Obese Patient

Michelle Olson, MD[a],*, Chris Pohl, MD[b]

KEYWORDS

- Obese • Body mass index • Percutaneous gastrostomy
- Procedure • Ultrasonography

BEDSIDE PROCEDURES

Although morbid obesity alone is not a contraindication to the performance of bedside procedures in the ICU, certain considerations must be made. Just as the performance of routine nursing tasks on morbidly obese patients requires additional staff and equipment,[1] so does safe bedside procedures. As with any procedure, attention should be given to equipment and proper ergonomics. When attending to morbidly obese patients in the ICU, additional assistance, as well as additional equipment, such as standing stools to improve access to patients across a wider bariatric bed, is likely required not only to move patients but also to aid in exposure.

PERCUTANEOUS ENDOSCOPIC GASTROSTOMY

Percutaneous endoscopic gastrostomy is widely used in the acute care setting to provide enteral feeding access and has several advantages over surgical gastrostomy.[2] During percutaneous endoscopic gastrostomy placement, it is common practice to transilluminate the abdominal wall with the endoscope and use finger indentation of the abdomen to determine correct placement. In morbidly obese patients, this can be a challenge because the thicker subcutaneous layer may make transillumination impossible and finger indentation unclear. In this case, additional maneuvers may be required. For example, a pre-existing surgical incision can be used to visualize the fascia and allow adequate transillumination for the procedure.[3]

---

[a] Department of General Surgery, Geisinger Medical Center, 100 North Academy Avenue, Danville, PA 17822, USA
[b] Department of Interventional Radiology, Geisinger Medical Center, 100 North Academy Avenue, Danville, PA 17822, USA
* Corresponding author.
E-mail address: mjreed17820@aol.com

Crit Care Clin 26 (2010) 665–668
doi:10.1016/j.ccc.2010.09.002
0749-0704/10/$ – see front matter © 2010 Elsevier Inc. All rights reserved.

The gastrostomy tube can then be tunneled subcutaneously to exit via a separate incision. Alternatively, the continuous aspiration technique can be used during gastric puncture, but with a thick abdominal wall it may be necessary to use a longer spinal needle with a smaller caliber guide wire.[4] With either method, preprocedure planning is necessary for success. Once the technical aspects of accomplishing the procedure have been addressed, the effect of the patient's abdominal pannus on the tube, specifically, whether or not the abdominal pannus will drag the tube caudally as the patient is moved from a supine to a more upright position. If this is not accounted for, the tube may cause necrosis of the abdominal wall from the pressure or may become completely dislodged. Use of a reverse Trendelenburg position during the procedure or before the procedure to mark proposed gastrostomy site may assist in improving tube placement.

PROCTOSCOPY AND SIGMOIDOSCOPY

Perianal inspection and proctoscopy or flexible sigmoidoscopy are also routine bedside procedures. Adequate lighting and exposure is necessary in any patient. In morbidly obese patients, positioning for these procedures often requires extra consideration. Not only is additional staff necessary to safely move patients into a lateral position but also consideration should be made of holding patients in that position. For this, large wedge pillows behind a patient's back may be helpful to allow adequate exposure to the perianal area. Additionally, the use of Velcro straps (as might be used in an operating room or endoscopy suite) can assist in stabilizing a patient. Adequate exposure of the perianal area can be difficult due to redundant tissues in the buttock. Better visualization can be achieved using tape straps (with appropriate caution to the condition of the patient's skin) or an assistant on the other side of the bed who can retract.

RADIOLOGIC PROCEDURES

Obese patients provide several special challenges for diagnostic and interventional radiology. Because of their increased diameter in any direction, the image quality of standard radiographs is reduced because of the increased scatter within a patient's body. Portable x-ray machines are limited in their penetrating often necessitating use of fixed installation radiographic equipment which usually lies outside the intensive care unit. Movement of the obese patient from the intensive care unit environment requires preparation and planning.

Imaging with ultrasound is more difficult because of the greater distance to be penetrated by the sound waves introduces significantly more image noise. Even with low-frequency, high-energy probes, sophisticated deep tissue interrogation, such as duplex, the image quality is limited. Optimizing patient positioning to achieve more effective acoustic windows is difficult, often requiring at least one or two patient care staff members to assist because patients are rarely able to reach or maintain awkward positions, such as a lateral decubitus position. Although increased manual pressure with the ultrasound probe may reduce the depth of overlying tissue, it also is a cause of rapid operator fatigue and in the long term accelerates work-related upper-extremity injuries. The benefit of ultrasound portability, however, makes the necessary additional patient care staff for the examination worthwhile.

CT and MRI are commonly limited by the actual bore size of the equipment as well as the table weight limit. Over the past few years, equipment manufacturers have responded by increasing the aperture of the scanner up to 70 cm and improving table construction to support a patient weight of 600 lb. To move patients onto the imaging equipment, electrical ceiling track mounted lifts are available to reduce the risk of work-related injury to staff and allow for a safer patient transfer. With patient size may still result in significant artifact near the edges and entire image degradation. Software improvements often allow for improved image reconstruction in these situations. The x-ray tubes have also been modified to provide higher radiation output and to dissipate the tremendous amount of additionally generated heat more rapidly to allow for spiral CT imaging in the heavier patient.

Using large, flexible, wrap-around coils or simply just the body coil is an alternative to the dedicated examination or body part–specific coils, which are generally too small. In order, however, to optimally image an area of interest with as little artifact as possible, it is helpful to artificially constrict a patient's girth extrinsically with linen or multiple wide elastic binders before placing a patient into the CT or MRI scanner. For ventilated patients, this is unlikely to interfere significantly with effective ventilation, but freely breathing patients may experience difficulty breathing, limiting the usefulness of such an adjunct. Often in morbidly obese patients, even assuming the perfectly supine position limits the ventilatory capacity, resulting in oxygen desaturation. Continuous positive airway pressure or bilevel positive airway pressure during those examinations is a simple step to improve ventilation and, thereby, patient comfort.

RADIOGRAPHIC DRAINAGE PROCEDURES

Radiographic access to various body cavities has become more common. Drainage of abscesses, pleural effusions, biliary stenting and placement of gastric tubes are some of the most common procedures for the critical ill patient. In addition to the difficulty of visualizing a target with various image-guided drainage procedures, the destination is sometimes beyond the reach of many access needles. During drainage procedures, the lack of clearance around a patient entering the CT scan gantry makes incremental approach to the target collection difficult. To achieve access to deep-seated collections in addition to the guess-and-stab or the guidance arm technique, a nested approach of short, larger, and then progressively longer and thinner needles is followed by sequential dilation and then catheter placement. Due to the potentially deep-seated nature of a collection, catheters are often inserted the entire length in the obese patient. Although some catheters are available in longer lengths, most are not. At time of insertion, consideration needs to be given to the degree of tissue mobility of the access site during position changes (especially to the upright position) to ensure that there is enough additional length of the catheter to prevent displacing the catheter. Placing the catheter on reservoir suction and frequently irrigating the catheter speeds up resolution of the collection. Given the challenges with accessing such a collection, the catheter generally needs to be larger than for a standard-sized adult to ensure successful drainage. A follow-up scan to confirm resolution before catheter removal is important to dramatically reduce the need for redrainage. Diagnostic and therapeutic paracentesis and thoracentesis are better performed by image guidance given the sometimes extensive amount of overlying soft tissue. Although sonography gives the freedom from the constraining gantry, it is operator dependent and a more deep-seated target may be difficult to visualize. Although CT can be more definitive in target identification and guidance, the limited gantry diameter can make a stepwise approach difficult. Placing patients off center into the gantry is helpful in identifying the skin entry site and gives slightly more room on the approach side while appropriately sacrificing image quality on the opposite side.

In summary, the obese critically ill patient can pose significant obstacles to common bedside and radiographic procedures. However with preparation, adequate staff and size appropriate equipment, these procedures can be done safely in these patients.

REFERENCES

1. Muir M, Heese GA, McLean D, et al. Handling of the bariatric patient in critical care: a case study of lessons learned. Crit Care Nurs Clin North Am 2007;19: 223–40.
2. Bankhead RR, Fisher CA, Rolandelli RH. Gastrostomy tube placement outcomes: comparison of surgical, endoscopic and laparoscopic methods. Nutr Clin Pract 2005;20:607–12.
3. Minocha A, Chotiprasidhi P, Elmajian D. PEG using a preexisting abdominal surgical incision in an obese patient with situs inversus. Gastrointest Endosc 1999;50:128.
4. Karhadkar A, Naini P, Dutta S. PEG-tube placement in a patient with extreme obesity: overcoming the technical challenges. Gastrointest Endosc 2007;65: 731–3.

Tracheostomy in Critical Ill Morbidly Obese

Michael Clark, MD[a], Scott Greene, DO[a],
Mary Jane Reed, MD, FCCM, FCCP[b],*

KEYWORDS

• Tracheostomy • Obese patients • Obstructive sleep apnea

TRACHEOTOMY IN THE OBESE PATIENT

Morbidly obese patients have a much higher incidence of obstructive sleep apnea (OSA) and also have altered respiratory physiology, including decreased respiratory compliance and increased airway resistance. Morbidly obese patients with ventilatory-dependent respiratory failure (VDRF) are more difficult to wean and extubate. Both OSA and VDRF are common indications of a tracheotomy in this patient population. Although there is a clear benefit to tracheotomy in obese patients with OSA and VDRF, this must be weighed against the increased surgical morbidity and mortality resulting from the patient's obesity. The 30-day postoperative mortality rate for a tracheotomy in the morbidly obese has been shown to be as high as 29%. With an elevated body mass index, the increased submental and anterior cervical adipose tissue not only adds to the difficulty of the surgical procedure but also leads to a size discrepancy and curvature mismatch between the tracheotomy tube and the stoma. Standard-sized tubes typically are too short and too curved. Modified tracheotomy tubes are available that are longer and more flexible, and although these tubes may fit properly, the longer tracheotomy track, as well as greater collapse of the stoma due to the anterior cervical adipose, complicates postoperative care, including tracheotomy tube changes. With a greater length of the tracheotomy tract, there is an increase risk of granulation tissue, bleeding from raw surfaces, and infection. The greatest concern of the longer track comes in the first couple weeks after surgery due to increased risk of decanulation, increased difficulty in replacing the track tube due to collapse of the stoma, and, therefore, increased risk of death.[1–3]

Alteration of a standard tracheotomy procedure should be considered to improve the fit of a standard tracheotomy tube or even a custom tube. A patient's neck should

---

[a] Department of Otolaryngology, Geisinger Medical Center, 100 North Academy Avenue, Danville, PA 17822, USA
[b] Departments of General Surgery and Critical Care Medicine, Geisinger Medical Center, Temple University Medical School, 100 North Academy Avenue, Mail Code: 20-37, Danville, PA 17822, USA
* Corresponding author.
E-mail address: Mjreed17820@aol.com

Crit Care Clin 26 (2010) 669–670
doi:10.1016/j.ccc.2010.09.003   **criticalcare.theclinics.com**

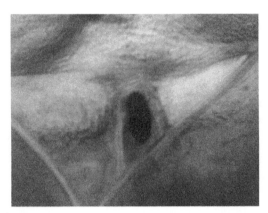

Fig. 1. Skin-lined stoma.

be carefully examined in the upright position to determine if either or both the submental adipose and anterior cervical adipose tissue need to be removed. The goal is to prevent the submental fat pad from draping over the proposed tracheostomy site and obstructing the orifice. Removal of both the submental fat pad and anterior cervial adipose tissue allows for a skin-lined stoma (**Fig. 1**) that decreases complications in postoperative care and the possibility of removing the tracheostomy tube without concern for stoma collapse long term.

Percutaneous tracheostomy has been safely performed in morbidly obese ventilator dependent patients.[4] Anterior fat pad depth, inability to hyperextend the neck, and need to adjust operator techniques, such as transillumination, should be considered. As with open tracheostomy, attention to submental fat pad drape in the upright position and adequate length of tracheostomy tube is imperative.

REFERENCES

1. Darrat I, Yaremchuk K. Early mortality rate of morbidly obese patients after tracheotomy. Laryngoscope 2008;118:2125–8.
2. Eliachar I, Zohar S, Golz A, et al. Permanent tracheostomy. Head Neck Surg 1984; 7:99–103.
3. Gross ND, Cohen JI, Andersen PE, et al. 'Defatting' tracheotomy in morbidly obese patients. Laryngoscope 2002;112:1940–4.
4. Mansharamani N, Koziel H. Safety of bedside percutaneous dilational tracheostomy in obese patients in the ICU. Chest 2000;117:1426–9.

Nutrition in Critically Ill Obese Patients

Naeem Raza, MD[a], Peter N. Benotti, MD[b],
Christopher D. Still, DO[c],*

KEYWORDS

- Enteral nutrition • Hypocalroic • High protein feed
- Permissive underfeeding • Obesity

Key points

Nutritional support is a vital part of care in critically ill obese patients.

Enteral nutrition is always the first choice if the gastrointestinal (GI) tract is functioning.

Overfeeding can lead to fluid overload, hyperglycemia, hepatic steatosis, and the need for prolonged ventilator support.

Hypocaloric, high protein nutritional feeding might have a role in critically ill obese patients.

Recently, there has been a growth in the prevalence of obesity, especially in developed countries. The standard definition of obesity is a body mass index (BMI) of 30 or more, calculated as the weight in kilograms divided by the height in meters squared. During the past 20 years, there has been a dramatic increase in obesity in the United States to the extent that it is now considered an epidemic. According to the Centers for Disease Control and Prevention, in 2008, only 1 state (Colorado) had a prevalence of obesity less than 20%. The prevalence of obesity in 32 states was equal to or greater than 25%; 6 of these states (Alabama, Mississippi, Oklahoma, South Carolina, Tennessee, and West Virginia) had a prevalence of obesity equal to or greater than 30%.

Timely assessment of nutritional needs is essential to improve the outcome of patients in the intensive care units (ICUs). A significant delay in feeding critically ill patients not only leads to increased risk of malnourishment but also results in delayed wound healing, increased risk of infections, and increased hospital length of stay.[1,2] The rate of catabolism is much higher than anabolic activity in critically ill patients.[3,4]

[a] Department of Gastroenterology and Nutrition, Geisinger Medical Center, MC 21-11, 100 North Academy Avenue, Danville, PA 17822, USA
[b] Department of Surgery, St Francis Medical Center, Trenton, NJ, USA
[c] Department of Gastroenterology and Nutrition, Center for Nutrition and Weight Management, Geisinger Obesity Institute, Geisinger Health System, MC 21-11, 100 North Academy Avenue, Danville, PA 17822, USA
* Corresponding author.
E-mail address: cstill@geisinger.edu

Crit Care Clin 26 (2010) 671–678
doi:10.1016/j.ccc.2010.08.004
0749-0704/10/$ – see front matter © 2010 Published by Elsevier Inc.

With the advantage of better nutrition in the form of adequate calories and protein during the recovery phase, this balance tilts toward an anabolic state, when anabolic activity exceeds catabolism. On the other hand, overfeeding obese patients also leads to medical complications. The appropriate balance of caloric and nutritional support for critically ill obese patients continues to be a clinical challenge.

Obesity is a risk factor for many serious medical diseases, such as cardiac diseases, stroke, diabetes, obesity-hypoventilation syndrome, and fatty liver disease. During a stay in the ICU, timely initiation of appropriate nutrition is a critical component of medical care. There are many advantages for providing nutrition during the care of severe catabolic state in the critical care unit. As a general rule, the enteral route is the preferred choice for providing nutrition. Although critically ill obese patients need special medical and nutritional care as do nonobese patients in the ICU, there are some differences mentioned in the literature about the initiation, routes, and nature of nutritional support. This article reviews the norms of nutritional care in critically ill obese patients and the differences between these patients and those with a normal BMI.

ENTERAL NUTRITION

The timing of initiation of nutrition and routes of choice are essential components of nutritional support. Enteral nutrition is a method of providing nutrition through the intestinal route.[5,6] A feeding tube can be introduced into the intestinal tract orally or directly into the stomach and small bowel. Evidence from many studies and meta-analyses has shown advantages to the early use of enteral nutrition in the form of decreased infection rate and reduced mortality.

The first step before initiating nutrition is to decide about the best available route to access the GI tract. Feeding tubes may be inserted through the orogastric or nasogastric route. Feeding tubes have the important features of being smaller and easier to maneuver because of their flexibility when compared with the tubes used for gastric decompression. These tubes can be easily placed at the bedside. Some types of tubes are better equipped for ease of intubation and feeding. Corflo feeding tubes has printed centimeter markings to aid bedside placement and check migration. These tubes have a weighted end required for stylet insertion. The stylets allow flow-through, which helps to flush, auscultate, and aspirate during the insertion. The position of the tube needs to be confirmed radiologically. After confirmation of the tube's position, the stylet is removed before initiating feeding.

Patients with a normal gut function and the need for long-term enteral feeding should be considered for placement of a percutaneous endoscopic feeding tube. Other indications for the use of percutaneous feeding tubes in the ICU include mechanical obstruction in the oropharyngeal or esophageal structures. These tubes are placed directly into the stomach or small bowel. Tubes can be placed by different methods (endoscopically, radiologically, or surgically). The decision to place these tubes requires complex reasoning and consent from the patients or their families. The endoscopic technique is the procedure of first choice and can be performed at the bedside. If this method fails, tube placement by interventional radiology under fluoroscopic guidance is usually considered. A surgical approach is considered if the patient warrants an abdominal operation for other reasons.

Endoscopic placement of gastrostomy tubes may be challenging in morbidly obese patients. During percutaneous endoscopic gastrostomy (PEG) tube placements, the lack of transillumination and inability to indicate the site of placement by finger indentation are considered absolute contraindications to the procedure by many gastroenterologists, although there are some studies in the literature to challenge this. Stewart and Hagan[7] reported that 60 of 62 patients (97%) had successful deployment of PEG tubes without transillumination. In another study, Minocha and colleagues[8] suggested another technique, in which patients had surgical incisions to open the subcutaneous layer of fat and visualize the transilluminated area better. Most of these methods are not practiced as frequently as the standard techniques in morbidly obese patients. In these patients, failures in PEG tube placement typically lead to radiologically guided or surgical methods.

In 2005, Bankhead and colleagues[9] published a study of 91 patients who had gastrostomy tube placement by 1 of the 3 techniques. Major reasons for feeding tube placement were ventilator-dependent respiratory failure, dysphagia, and head and neck cancer. Among these 91 patients, 23 had PEG tube placements, 39 received laparoscopic procedures, and 29 had open surgical techniques for feeding tube placement. One expected difference was the time needed for the procedure. The bedside placement of PEG tubes required a minimum of 30 minutes when compared with the laparoscopic technique (48 minutes) and the surgical method (68 minutes). Failure of insertion was higher by the laparoscopic method (3 patients) followed by PEG tube insertion (1 patient). The laparoscopic technique was also associated with more complications, such as cellulitis, bleeding, and serous drainage, whereas open surgical techniques had delays in the start of feeding.[9] In the conclusion, authors cite percutaneuous endoscopic placement of gastrostomy tube as a treatment of choice.

Bochicchio and colleagues[10] conducted a brief study, in which only 6 patients with a BMI greater than 60 had successful PEG tube placement by an experienced surgical endoscopist using the pull technique. Overall, the number of patients was too small to draw a conclusion for guidelines. In some cases (eg, necrotizing pancreatitis) post pyloric feeding tubes are used to provide nutrition. Placement of these tubes can be achieved by bedside technique. Endoscopic technique, radiological methods with fluoroscopic guidance or surgical approach are other means to assist in placement of these tubes. Insertion of this feeding tube through oral routes can be blind and done at the bedside. The aim is to place the terminal end of the tube beyond the pylorus in the small bowel. The position of the tube needs to be confirmed radiologically before starting feeding. These tubes can also be placed under direct vision endoscopically.

The next step after establishing and confirming access is to decide about the types of nutrition to provide for critically ill obese patients. Nutritional formulas differ with respect to calories, osmolarity, protein content, electrolytes, and other contents. The standard enteral nutritional formula consists of isotonic, lactose-free, nonhydrolyzed protein contents, a mixture of simple and complex carbohydrates, and long-chain fatty acids. Normally, the ratio of nonprotein calories to nitrogen content is around 150:1. Some critically ill patients may require concentrated nutrition because of the need for volume restriction. Concentrated feedings are difficult to tolerate and can lead to dumping syndrome and diarrhea. The main difference between standard and concentrated formulas is in osmolarity and caloric content. The concentrated formulas are hyperosmolar and hypercaloric.

SPECIAL NUTRITIONAL CONSIDERATIONS IN CRITICALLY ILL OBESE PATIENTS

Nutritional assessment is the first step in providing nutritional therapy in critically ill patients. A stepwise approach enables the care provider to optimize therapy. To understand the nutritional and metabolic profile of each patient one should measure the height in centimeters, weight in kilograms, basal energy expenditures in kilocalories per day, actual weight as a percentage of ideal weight, and triceps fold size. A review of the laboratory test results, including levels of serum albumin, prealbumin, and serum transferrin, and the assessment of nitrogen balance is essential.[11]

Understanding the concept of nitrogen balance is an important step in assessing a nutritional regimen for all patients, especially the critically ill obese patient. Nitrogen balance is defined as follows:

Nitrogen balance = Nitrogen input − Nitrogen output

Blackburn and colleagues have mentioned the following formula for calculation of nitrogen balance at the bedside[11]:

Nitrogen balance = (Protein intake/6.25) − (Urinary urea nitrogen + 4)

Nitrogen intake is assessed by measuring the protein intake per day in grams and dividing this by 6.25. On the other hand, it is difficult to calculate nitrogen output because of miscellaneous nitrogen loss (GI and insensible), which adds to urinary nitrogen loss. Urinary nitrogen loss is calculated in a 24-hour urine specimen. A positive nitrogen balance indicates an anabolic state, whereas a negative balance indicates catabolism. Positive nitrogen balance is achieved by increasing protein intake or energy intake. Dickerson and colleagues[12] has reported that net protein anabolism can be achieved in obese patients with high protein intake combined with low caloric intake. The other possible ways to increase nitrogen balance are to add more protein and decrease caloric intake.[13] An increased intake of hypercaloric food, more than the body needs, leads to the accumulation of fat mass. For obese patients, a low-caloric, high protein intake can promote nitrogen equilibrium and positive nitrogen balance without adding body fat, which is very important in critically ill patients who typically have an increased rate of negative nitrogen balance in the form of catabolism.

HYPOCALORIC, HIGH PROTEIN FEEDING IN OBESE PATIENTS

In the past, there was a trend to feed critically ill patients a hypercaloric metabolic diet. Several studies reported undesirable outcomes among these patients in the form of increased carbohydrate overload and respiratory complications leading to prolonged mechanical ventilation.[14–17] These observations led to an emphasis on balancing the protein and energy needs of both obese and nonobese hospitalized patients. One noteworthy observation is that obese patients require reduced caloric intake to prevent accumulation of body fat. There are different studies regarding hypocaloric feeding with reduced or normal protein intake in obese patients. The advantages of hypocaloric, high protein nutritional supportover higher calorie diets are better metabolic equilibrium, achievement of nitrogen balance, loss of adipose tissue, and preservation of lean body muscle mass.

Dickerson and colleagues[12] conducted a small study on 13 postoperative obese patients to evaluate the clinical outcome associated with a hypocaloric, high protein parenteral nutrition. This study was a prospective one of critically ill obese patients on hypocaloric (881 kcal/d), high protein (2.13 ± 0.59 g/kg) total parenteral nutrition. The outcome was measured in the form of nitrogen balance and by follow-up of wound and fistula healing. Results not only showed positive nitrogen balance in 8 of the 13 patients but also revealed promising clinical outcomes including closure of fistulas and complete tissue healing of wounds and abscess cavities. The investigators concluded that hypocaloric, high protein nutritional support is associated with nitrogen equilibrium and good clinical outcomes in critically ill obese patients.[12]

Another study reported by Burge and colleagues[18] did not reveal significant outcomes with a similar feeding strategy. The study evaluated 16 critically ill obese patients. In this study, hypocaloric, high protein nutritional support was compared with normocaloric, high protein support. No significant difference was noted in nitrogen balance.

Choban and colleagues[19] performed a randomized double-blind trial to compare hypocaloric parenteral nutrition with higher caloric parenteral nutrition among obese patients. They randomly assigned 30 obese patients with a BMI of 35 to a hypoenergetic parenteral regimen or to an isonitrogenous normoenergetic formula (control group). Nitrogen balance was determined on day 0 and weekly. The total energy intake was 57 ± 12 kJ in the hypoenergetic group compared with 94 ± 21 kJ in the control group. Protein intake was the same. In this study, the mean net nitrogen balance was not different for the 2 groups. There was also no significant weight change between the 2 groups.[19]

Hypocaloric, high protein enteral feeding was studied among 42 critically ill obese patients by Dickerson and colleagues.[20] In this study, the patients were randomized to receive a high caloric intake or a low caloric intake, with a mean protein intake of 1.9 g/kg ideal body weight (IBW) and 1.5 g/kg IBW, respectively. Although this study did not reveal significant differences in the nitrogen balance at weeks 1 and 2, patients with hypocaloric, high protein intake showed a decrease in the length of ICU stay (18.5 ± 9.9 days vs 28.5 ± 16.1 days $P<.03$). Other key findings included a trend toward decreased days on ventilator and antibiotics among patients in the hypocaloric, high protein intake group.[20]

The analysis based on a review of the literature on critically ill obese patients regarding the use of high protein hypoenergetic nutrition is promising. However, the validity of these results requires further randomized double-blind studies.

Some studies have shown less-effective outcomes with hypocaloric parenteral nutrition. One retrospective study by Liu and colleagues[21] compared 2 groups of obese patients. The first group included patients younger than 60 years and the other group consisted of patients older than 60 years. Energy intake was divided in the 2 groups based on the IBW. Patients weighing more than 150% of the IBW were given 60% of the total required calories. The other group of patients weighing between 120% and 150% of the IBW were given 75% of the total caloric requirement. All patients were provided with 1.5 g/kg of protein. There was a difference in the nitrogen balance between the 2 groups. The group younger than 60 years had a nitrogen balance of $+3.4 \pm 3.9$ g/d compared with the group older than 60 years, which had a nitrogen balance of $+0.2 \pm 5$ g/d ($P = .06$). This result is not significant, and also there was no difference in clinical outcome between the 2 groups.

Some researchers have hypothesized that the obese patient has impaired fat oxidative metabolism. This idea was extracted from a study in which net fat oxidation rate was evaluated by indirect calorimetry and measurement of glycerol oxidation in obese patients. Comparisons were made with the values for the nonobese patients. The study was conducted for 2 to 4 days before placing these patients on nutritional support. In this study, the obese group showed a decrease in net fat oxidation rate compared with the nonobese group ($P<.001$). Whether this is a transient clinical condition before starting hypercaloric, high protein feeding is not confirmed. There is further need for study in a larger group of patients.[22]

In conclusion, hypocaloric, high protein nutritional support has a role among critically ill obese patients in increasing positive nitrogen balance and improving clinical outcome without adding any deleterious side effects. Hypocaloric support groups also show better carbohydrate control. A cautious approach should be used in providing this hypocaloric, high protein nutritional support in patients older than 60 years as suggested by Liu and colleagues.[21]

FLUID STATUS

Fluid balance is an important consideration in critically ill obese patients. The risk of volume overload is high in these patients because they often receive standard nutritional support with additional intravenous fluids in the setting of coexisting conditions such as cardiac, liver, and renal diseases. Concentrated nutrition in patients at risk of fluid overload may be a better alternative in this situation. Concentrated nutrition, however, may be difficult to tolerate and is associated with the risk of diarrhea and dumping syndrome. This risk of intolerance is more significant for patients fed with concentrated postpyloric feedings.

OVERFEEDING

Although undernourishment of critically ill obese patients increases the risk of unwanted medical consequences, overfeeding can also be equally detrimental to recovery. Obese patients frequently have difficulty weaning from ventilators.[23] Overfeeding increases carbon dioxide production, increasing minute ventilatory demands and prolonging ventilator length of stay. Aggressive feeding in obese patients with baseline fatty liver and nonalcoholic steatohepatitis leads to more hepatic fat accumulation and an increase in hepatic dysfunction. Other adverse outcomes of overfeeding consist of immune suppression, depressed renal function, and poor control of glucose levels.[23]

PERMISSIVE UNDERFEEDING IN CRITICALLY ILL OBESE PATIENTS

Because of the demonstrated problems associated with overfeeding critically ill patients, there is an interest in the use of permissive underfeeding to minimize the complications of overfeeding. In a review of permissive underfeeding, Malone[24] has reported potential mechanisms for the beneficial effects of underfeeding, including reduced hyperglycemia by limiting carbohydrate intake and decreased production of inflammatory mediators such as free radicals and cytokines. Other beneficial effects of underfeeding include the decrease in carbon dioxide production as reported in many studies and a decrease in respiratory work.[24] There are a few studies in laboratory animals supporting this evidence. In these studies, groups with restricted diets demonstrated decreased oxidant production and showed lower mortality compared with groups with normal intake.

GLUCOSE

Obese patients also have a risk of more fluid retention and glucose intolerance because of the stress of critical illness and the underlying insulin resistance. Increased carbohydrate overload due to hypercaloric nutritional support in these patients can cause respiratory complications leading to prolonged mechanical ventilation, accumulation of more body fat, and hepatic steatosis.[15,16] On the other hand, strict control of glucose levels (70 mg/dL–110 mg/dL) in critically ill surgical patients has been associated with improved morbidity and mortality.[25]

SUMMARY

Critically ill obese patients require timely nutrition in the ICU. Enteral nutrition is better than parenteral nutrition if the gut can tolerate. In obese patients, overfeeding and fluid overload should be avoided. Blood glucose levels should be monitored closely. Critically ill obese patients need to be assessed individually based on their caloric and protein needs, their clinical problems, and the goals for recovery. Hypocaloric, high protein nutritional feeding should be considered for the critically ill obese patient. This formula leads to fewer complications, positive nitrogen balance, and better clinical outcomes. Confirmation of these positive findings will require larger randomized double-blind trials.

REFERENCES

1. Marik PE, Zaloga GP. Early enteral nutrition in acutely ill patients: a systematic review. Crit Care Med 2001;29(12):2264–70.
2. Blackburn GL, Maini BS, Pierce EC Jr. Nutrition in the critically ill patient. Anesthesiology 1977;47(2):181–94.
3. Dabrowski GP, Rombeau JL. Practical nutritional management in the trauma intensive care unit. Surg Clin North Am 2000;80(3):921–32, x.
4. Beale RJ, Bryg DJ, Bihari DJ. Immunonutrition in the critically ill: a systematic review of clinical outcome. Crit Care Med 1999;27(12):2799–805.
5. Braunschweig CL, Levy P, Sheean PM, et al. Enteral compared with parenteral nutrition: a meta-analysis. Am J Clin Nutr 2001;74(4):534–42.
6. ASPEN Board of Directors and the Clinical Guidelines Task Force. Guidelines for the use of parenteral and enteral nutrition in adult and pediatric patients. JPEN J Parenter Enteral Nutr 2002;26(Suppl 1):1SA–138SA.
7. Stewart JA, Hagan P. Failure to transilluminate the stomach is not an absolute contraindication to PEG insertion. Endoscopy 1998;30(7):621–2.
8. Minocha A, Chotiprasidhi P, Elmajian DA. PEG using a preexisting abdominal surgical incision in an obese patient with situs inversus. Gastrointest Endosc 1999;50(1):128.
9. Bankhead RR, Fisher CA, Rolandelli RH. Gastrostomy placement outcomes: comparison of surgical, endoscopic, and laparoscopic methods. Nutr Clin Pract 2005;20(6):607–12.
10. Bochicchio GV, Guzzo JL, Scalea TM. Percutaneous endoscopic gastrostomy in the supermorbidly obese patient. JSLS 2006;10(4):409–13.
11. Blackburn GL, Bistrian BR, Maini BS, et al. Nutritional and metabolic assessment of the hospitalized patient. JPEN J Parenter Enteral Nutr 1977;1(1):11–22.
12. Dickerson RN, Rosato EF, Mullen JL. Net protein anabolism with hypocaloric parenteral nutrition in obese stressed patients. Am J Clin Nutr 1986;44(6): 747–55.
13. Elwyn DH. Nutritional requirements of adult surgical patients. Crit Care Med 1980; 8(1):9–20.
14. Robin AP, Askanazi J, Cooperman A, et al. Influence of hypercaloric glucose infusions on fuel economy in surgical patients: a review. Crit Care Med 1981;9(9): 680–6.
15. Delafosse B, Bouffard Y, Viale JP, et al. Respiratory changes induced by parenteral nutrition in postoperative patients undergoing inspiratory pressure support ventilation. Anesthesiology 1987;66(3):393–6.
16. Covelli HD, Black JW, Olsen MS, et al. Respiratory failure precipitated by high carbohydrate loads. Ann Intern Med 1981;95(5):579–81.
17. Askanazi J, Rosenbaum SH, Hyman AI, et al. Respiratory changes induced by the large glucose loads of total parenteral nutrition. JAMA 1980;243(14): 1444–7.

18. Burge JC, Goon A, Choban PS, et al. Efficacy of hypocaloric total parenteral nutrition in hospitalized obese patients: a prospective double-blind randomized trial. JPEN J Parenter Enteral Nutr 1994;18:203–7.

19. Choban PS, Burge JC, Scales D, et al. Hypoenergetic nutrition support in hospitalized obese patients: a simplified method for clinical application. Am J Clin Nutr 1997;66(3):546–50.

20. Dickerson RN, Boschert KJ, Kudsk KA, et al. Hypocaloric enteral tube feeding in critically ill obese patients. Nutrition 2002;18(3):241–6.

21. Liu KJ, Cho MJ, Atten MJ, et al. Hypocaloric parenteral nutrition support in elderly obese patients. Am Surg 2000;66(4):394–9 [discussion: 399–400].

22. Jeevanandam M, Young DH, Schiller WR. Obesity and the metabolic response to severe multiple trauma in man. J Clin Invest 1991;87(1):262–9.

23. Marik P, Varon J. The obese patient in the ICU. Chest 1998;113(2):492–8.

24. Malone AM. Permissive underfeeding: its appropriateness in patients with obesity, patients on parenteral nutrition, and non-obese patients receiving enteral nutrition. Curr Gastroenterol Rep 2007;9(4):317–22.

25. Van den Berghe G, Wilmer A, Milants I, et al. Intensive insulin therapy in mixed medical/surgical intensive care units: benefit versus harm. Diabetes 2006; 55(11):3151–9.

Pharmacotherapy in the Critically Ill Obese Patient

Charles J. Medico, PharmD, BCPS[a,b,*], Patrick Walsh, DO, FCCP[c,d]

KEYWORDS

- Pharmacotherapy • Obese • Dosing • Body weight

Dosing medications in the obese patient remains a challenge in spite of the fact that 34% of Americans are considered obese, a percentage that has doubled since 1980 according to the statistics of the Centers for Disease Control and Prevention. Premarketing drug studies rarely address obese patients proportionately with patients of a normal body mass index ([BMI] calculated as the weight in kilograms divided by height in meters squared). As a result of the disproportion of the size of patients included in these studies, manufacturers show bias because the studies are usually conducted in patients who are of normal BMI. In addition, when obese patients are included in the dosing studies of new medications, these patients usually constitute the minority of the study population. Furthermore, most drug studies using obese patients are conducted by independent researchers during the postmarketing period of medication study design.

The physiologic changes associated with obesity have a large impact on drug metabolism and distribution. Although drug absorption in obese people has shown to be unchanged,[1] drug excretion is increased in these people because of an increase in glomerular filtration rate (GFR).[2,3] Many medications used in the critically ill obese patient can be overdosed if actual body weight is used or underdosed if standard manufacturer dosing recommendations are used. Extrapolating standard manufacturer dosing recommendations to the obese critically ill patient can lead to drug

The authors had no financial support to disclose.

[a] Division of System Therapeutics and Critical Care Medicine, Geisinger Medical Center, 100 North Academy Avenue, Danville, PA 17822, USA

[b] Department of Pharmacy Practice, Wilkes University Nesbitt College of Pharmacy and Nursing, 84 West South Street, Wilkes-Barre, PA 18766, USA

[c] Division of Critical Care Medicine, Geisinger Medical Center, 100 North Academy Avenue, Danville, PA 17822, USA

[d] Departments of Medicine and Surgery, Temple University School of Medicine, 3400 North Broad Street, Philadelphia, PA 19140, USA

* Corresponding author. System Therapeutics, Geisinger Medical Center, 100 North Academy Avenue, Danville, PA 17822.

E-mail address: cjmedico@geisinger.edu

Crit Care Clin 26 (2010) 679–688
doi:10.1016/j.ccc.2010.07.003
0749-0704/10/$ – see front matter © 2010 Elsevier Inc. All rights reserved.

criticalcare.theclinics.com

toxicity or treatment failure. The lack of dosing information in the morbidly obese patient causes many practitioners to fear the consequences of toxicity. This fear has led to the avoidance of some drugs in this population, including drotrecogin alfa and low–molecular-weight heparin.

The volume of distribution (Vd) of most drugs is primarily dependent on the lipophilicity of the drug.[1,4,5] In general, lipophilic medications are associated with higher volumes of distribution, which usually require total body weight (TBW) dosing. In contrast, hydrophilic medications are associated with lower volumes of distribution, which usually require ideal body weight (IBW) or adjusted body weight dosing.

It is imperative to use drug monitoring and clinical pharmacists to aid in the dosing of the critically ill obese patient when available. In many studies, the aid of well-trained clinical pharmacists involved in the direct care of the critically ill patient has been shown to reduce mortality, costs, duration of stay, readmission rates, and bleeding complications while improving clinical outcomes.[6–9] The drug serum level, activated partial thromboplastin time (APTT), international normalized ratio, heparin Xa assay results, hemoglobin level, or serum creatinine level can be helpful to guide appropriate drug dosing or to identify toxicity in the obese patient. Expected clinical outcomes should also be carefully monitored, such as resolution of fever, sterilization of infected fluids, resolution of pulmonary infiltrates, reduction of heart rate, pain control, agitation control, or liberation from ventilator support.

Despite the publication of many retrospective studies analyzing the pharmacokinetics of medications in the obese patient, it is still difficult to find large prospective trials with outcomes data in obese patients. The following drug dosing recommendations are made based on the drug properties and the literature available, assuming normal renal and hepatic function. Obviously, the intent of any recommendation or guideline is to support good clinical judgment.

ENOXAPARIN

As some investigators have previously described, there is evidence to support the use of enoxaparin in morbidly obese people using actual body weight for both prophylaxis and treatment without a capped dose.[10–14] A treatment dose of 1 mg/kg actual body weight subcutaneously for every 12 hours with a goal heparin Xa assay of 0.6 to 1 U/mL drawn 4 hours after at least the third dose has been suggested in a review of the literature.[11,13,14]

Manufacturer's recommendation for prophylaxis dosing, 30 mg subcutaneously for every 12 hours or 40 mg subcutaneously daily, may not be appropriate for the morbidly obese person because these recommendations are made without an adequate obese population. Studies concerning venous thromboembolism (VTE) prevention in obese patients with medical illnesses further confirmed that standard fixed dosing may not achieve heparin Xa assay results within the suggested VTE prophylactic goal of 0.2 to 0.4 U/mL.[10,15,16] Although some studies have recommended an enoxaparin dose of 40 mg every 12 hours subcutaneously for VTE prophylaxis,[15] others have suggested a dose of 60 mg every 12 hours subcutaneously.[16,17] Both of these recommendations have led to inconsistent results by causing underdosing and overdosing in some patients, respectively. An individual, patient-specific, weight-based regimen for the prevention of VTE with enoxaparin makes the most clinical sense for morbidly obese patients.[10,12,14] In one small study, a weight-based dose of 0.5 mg/kg actual body weight subcutaneously for every 24 hours was shown to prevent VTE safely. In the same study, this regimen also consistently achieved heparin Xa assay results in the prophylactic goal range of 0.2 to 0.4 U/mL when drawn 4 hours after at least the third dose.[10]

HEPARIN

Although heparin has been available since 1936, many controversies remain 75 years later as to which weight (total vs adjusted vs ideal) to use when initiating intravenous heparin for the treatment of thromboembolic disease in the obese patient. A secondary dosing controversy also revolves around dose capping versus noncapped dosing. In the absence of good dosing studies involving critically ill obese patients, some best practice conclusions can be made about heparin dosing based on the published literature and pharmacodynamics of heparin.

Although obese patients have increased vasculature and blood volume, adipose tissue has much lesser vasculature and blood volume than lean tissue. The Vd of heparin is dependent on blood volume and is poorly distributed into adipose tissue. It is not appropriate to use IBW dosing and dose capping for weight-based dosing in the obese patient because the extravasculature and blood volume of obese patients would be omitted, leading to underdosing in patients who would then be at risk for clot progression, recurrence of thromboembolic events, and death.[18–28]

In addition, morbidly obese patients who are dosed based on actual body weight are at risk of overanticoagulation and bleeding because of the inclusion of adipose tissue at the dose in which heparin is poorly distributed.[22,23,25,27] A large study by Anand and colleagues[26] noted a 7% increase in major bleeding for every 10-second increase in the APTT. Furthermore, the GUSTO-IIB (Global Use of Strategies to Open Occluded Coronary Arteries in Acute Coronary Syndromes) study showed that a prolonged APTT at 6 hours increased the risk of moderate to severe bleeding.[26] Although supratherapeutic APTT has been shown to play a role in bleeding risk, it has also been determined that a patient's individual characteristics such as age older than 75 years, recent surgery, alcoholism, liver disease, trauma, diabetes, cancer, treated hypertension, cerebrovascular disease, renal disease, and concomitant treatment with other antiplatelet medications are the major risk factors for determining the bleeding risk.[26]

Because actual body weight dosing often yields overanticoagulation and IBW dosing or dose capping can produce subtherapeutic results, adjusted body weight dosing is becoming more attractive for the obese patient. Adjusted body weight dosing without dose capping should take into account the increased vasculature and blood volume of the obese patient while omitting the adipose tissue weight, which makes the most clinical sense.[24,27]

The adjusted body weight may be determined by

Adjusted body weight (kg) = IBW + 0.4 × (actual body weight − IBW)

Men: IBW (kg) = 50 + 2.3 × (height>60 in)

Women: IBW (kg) = 45.5 + 2.3 × (height>60 in)

For VTE prophylaxis some literature suggests[27,29]:

For BMI <50 kg/m^2, heparin 5000 U subcutaneously every 8 hours

For BMI ≥50 kg/m^2, heparin 7500 U subcutaneously every 8 hours

DROTRECOGIN ALFA ACTIVATED

Many clinicians have restricted the use of drotrecogin alfa to patients who weigh less than 135 kg. This practice parallels the exclusion criteria of the PROWESS

(Recombinant Human Activated Protein C Worldwide Evaluation in Severe Sepsis) trial.[30] Until 2005, there had been an uncertainty regarding the pharmacokinetics, pharmacodynamics, and safety of drotrecogin alfa when used in patients weighing more than 135 kg. A study conducted in 2005 by Levy and colleagues[31] showed that the kinetics and safety of drotrecogin alfa are not affected by dosing based on actual body weight, with no dosing cap and no weight restrictions up to 227 kg.

ARGATROBAN

Argatroban is a direct thrombin inhibitor, which is predominantly hepatically metabo-lized. The metabolism of this drug increases linearly with actual body weight.[32,33] Current manufacturer recommendations are to dose argatroban based on actual body weight up to 140 kg.[32] Furthermore, a study performed by Hursting and Jang[34] concluded that actual body weight, with a BMI up to 50.9 kg/m^2, should be used for argatroban dosing during percutaneous coronary intervention. Another retro-spective study by Rice and colleagues[35] concluded that actual body weight dosing led to no differences in the intensity of anticoagulation, clinical outcomes, and thrombotic risk in obese patients with heparin-induced thrombocytopenia (HIT) or presumed HIT when compared with nonobese patients with the same condition. However, like other argatroban studies, critically ill patients seem to require a reduced initial dosing of 1 μg/kg/min (even less with hepatic impairment), which is half of the dose suggested by manufacturer dosing guidelines.[35,36] Dosing adjustments should be made based on APTT monitoring.

CEPHALOSPORINS

These compounds are hydrophilic in nature with limited solubility in adipose tissue. Although little change for Vd in obesity is suspected, fat contains 30% water and leads to a substantially higher Vd in the obese patient. Both plasma volume and lean body mass are increased in obese patients when compared with matched controls based on sex and height, contributing to the increase in Vd.[37] In one study, the Vd for cefo-taxime was increased by 42% to 68%. However, the investigators did not think that the clinical relevance was sufficient enough to recommend change in dose. They do suggest that standardized dosing may be possible if targeted on the basis of the body surface area (BSA).[38]

Cefazolin is widely used as a prophylactic agent in a variety of surgical procedures, and it was studied in obese patients undergoing surgery. One group of normal weight patients and 2 groups of extremely obese patients (BMI ≥46) were studied. The groups received a single 1-g (normal weight), 1-g (obese), or 2-g (obese) dose of cefa-zolin, and the respective serum levels at incision time were 110.5 ± 18.9 μg, 65.2 ± 15 μg, and 127 ± 16.3 μg (P<.001). The serum concentrations in morbidly obese patients who received the 2-g dose were similar to those in the normal weight control group that were given the 1-g dose, whereas a 50% lower concentration resulted in obese patients who were given the 1-g dose.

Compared with historic controls, the rate of infections at the wound site was decreased from 16.5% to 5.6% (P<.3) and it was concluded that the 2-g dose should be used in obese patients.[39]

While using cephalosporins, it is therefore prudent to double the dose or adjust it according to the BSA to produce serum concentrations similar to that in normal weight patients, especially for life-threatening infections.[40]

PENICILLINS

A case report of a man with a BMI greater than 50 kg/m^2 who was treated with piper-acillin/tazobactam (Zosyn), 3.375 g every 4 hours, for cellulitis with positive wound cultures for group A and B *Streptococcus* and *Pseudomonas aeruginosa* revealed substantial differences in pharmacokinetic parameters compared with those in normal weight historic controls. The Vd was 54.3 L versus 12.7 L (normal weight), serum steady concentration 39.8 mg/L versus 123.6 mg/L, and half-life 0.6 hours versus 1.4 hours for piperacillin. The 8:1 ratio of piperacillin to tazobactam was maintained in this instance. Serum concentrations for piperacillin at 30 minutes, 2 hours, and 4 hours were 242 mg/L, 34.6 mg/L, and 5.1 mg/L, and *P aeruginosa* is considered susceptible to piperacillin/tazobactam if the minimal inhibitory concentration (MIC) is 64 mg/L or less.[41] It is currently recommended that serum concentrations are main-tained above the MIC for at least 50% of the dosing interval and outcomes may be improved as the proportion of the dosing interval increases above 4.3 times the MIC.[42]

This study suggests the need for further investigation to clarify the dosing regimen for obese patients. A dose adjustment or continuous infusion should be considered for *P aeruginosa* infections with a higher MIC (>16).

Limited data are available for other penicillins. However, as a class, penicillins have similar pharmacokinetic profiles, suggesting that an increased dose may be beneficial in obese patients.

CARBAPENEMS

A study comparing the pharmacokinetics of ertapenem in 30 healthy volunteers exam-ined these patients in 3 groups of 10 according to weight, normal (BMI = 18.5–24.9 kg/m^2), class I-II obesity (BMI = 30–39.9 kg/m^2), and class III obesity (BMI $\geq$40 kg/m^2). Significant differences were noted in serum concentration between the obese and normal weight groups.

The area under the concentration curve in the normal weight group was significantly larger than that in the class II and class III obese patients. Carbapenem bactericidal activity is time dependent. Thus, the duration of the dosing interval in which the serum levels are above the MIC (ƒT>MIC) is important for maximal bactericidal effect. All 3 groups had a 90% probability of maintaining serum concentrations above the MIC (ƒT>MIC) for more than 20% of the dosing interval assuming an MIC less than or equal to 0.25 µg/ml. The same MIC (ƒT>MIC) target for an MIC less than or equal to 0.5 µg/ml could be achieved in only 90% of the normal weight subjects and none of the obese patients studied.[43]

A higher dose of ertapenem should be considered in obese patients who are infected with organisms having MICs greater than 0.25 µg/ml to 0.5 µg/ml because the standard 1-g dose may not provide an adequate duration of exposure for concen-trations above the MIC.[43]

OXAZOLIDINONES

Linezolid pharmacokinetics was studied in 7 obese patients (>50% heavier than calcu-lated IBW) with cellulitis, and the results demonstrated an overall decrease in serum levels at all dosing intervals. All patients were at steady state after receiving multiple doses (range 3–12, median 7) before the collection of serum samples for the trough and at time intervals of 1 and 6 hours after the morning dose of linezolid. The mean concentrations were 4.2 µg/ml, 12.5 µg/ml, and 7.2 µg/ml for the respective time inter-vals mentioned, and the serum inhibitory titers were sufficient with the exception of one strain of methicillin-resistant *Staphylococcus aureus* ([MRSA], MIC of 4 µg/ml). Cultures from the patients yielded 3 isolates of *S aureus* ([MRSA], MIC 1, 2, 4 µg/ml) and one each of *Enterococcus faecium* vancomycin-resistant enterococci (MIC 2 µg/ml), *Bacteroides fragilis* (MIC 2 µg/ml), and *Peptostreptococcus magnus* (MIC 1 µg/ml). Serum concentration over time in relation to the MIC for the organism is most important for maximal effect.[44]

In a murine model, the ratio of the area under the curve at 24 hours (AUC_{24}) to the MIC of 83, which represents the concentration over time in relation to the MIC, provided an adequate bacteriostatic effect against *Staphylococcus*.[40] The pharmacokinetic results of this study indicate that standard dosing should provide a bacteriostatic effect (AUC_{24}/MIC) ratio of 83 against *S aureus* with MICs less than or equal to 2 µg/ml. In vitro studies were used to test sera from the obese patients against the isolates listed, and the results demonstrated a prolonged (>12 hour) inhibitory activity for bacteria with MIC less than 2 µg/ml but not for the isolate with an MIC of 4 µg/ml. All patients received linezolid, 600 mg by mouth every 12 hours, and it was effective for the entire study group. Consideration for a dose increase may be prudent in patients with isolates exhibiting an MIC of 4 µg/ml.[45]

LIPOPEPTIDES

A single-dose pharmacokinetic study using daptomycin in 3 groups of volunteers who had normal weight, were moderately obese (BMI 25–39.9 kg/m^2), and were morbidly obese (BMI$\geq$40 kg/m^2) concludes that the dose of daptomycin should be based on TBW in obesity.[46] This dosing regimen increases daptomycin exposure (maximum concentration [C_{max}], AUC) by 25% and 30% and is considered safe and well tolerated when compared with earlier-collected safety data and trials.[46]

Another study comparing a daptomycin dose of 4 mg/kg TBW in 7 morbidly obese (BMI 46.2 $\pm$ 5.5 kg/m^2) and 7 normal weight subjects (BMI 21.8 $\pm$ 1.9 kg/m^2) also suggests that TBW dosing is appropriate. The TBW and Vd correlation was good compared with the poor correlation between IBW and Vd. The creatinine clearance determined by the Cockcroft-Gault equation using TBW overestimated the GFR, and the IBW provided an unbiased estimate of the GFR. This study demonstrated a higher C_{max} (60%) and AUC in morbidly obese patients than in normal weight subjects, which was different from the prior study. Future studies are required to provide information to improve dosing strategies for daptomycin in morbidly obese patients with chronic renal insufficiency.[47,48]

QUINOLONES

The pharmacokinetics of ciprofloxacin was studied in 17 moderately obese patients and 11 normal weight subjects. There was a significantly larger Vd in the obese, but when corrected for TBW, the Vd was significantly smaller in the obese patients. Based on the partial distribution of the drug into fat tissue, the investigators recommend adding 45% of excess weight to the IBW for dose calculations.[49] In a case report on a 226-kg patient who received ciprofloxacin, 800 mg intravenously every 12 hours, therapeutic serum concentrations were obtained at the given dose.[50]

VANCOMYCIN

Although the early use of vancomycin was associated with numerous adverse effects such as nephrotoxicity, ototoxicity, and infusion-related reactions, the recent cleaner formulations of vancomycin appears to be safer for patients. The current literature provides conflicting data to support nephrotoxicity and ototoxicity from vancomycin alone. The increasing incidence of serious MRSA infections in the critically ill makes vancomycin one of the most commonly prescribed antibiotics today. Unlike other drugs that lack information for obese patients, vancomycin remains one of the most widely studied antibiotics in the obese patient. In 2009, as a result of the information and data that the medical community has acquired over the long history of vancomycin use, the Society of Health-System Pharmacists, the Infectious Diseases Society of America, and the Society of Infectious Diseases Pharmacists published detailed consensus guidelines for dosing and monitoring of vancomycin in all patient populations, including the obese patient. According to these 3 organizations, vancomycin is to be dosed, 15 to 20 mg/kg actual body weight for every 8 to 12 hours, in all patient populations with good renal function. Further dosing adjustments should be made to achieve a goal steady-state trough level of 15 to 20 mg/L. For critically ill patients an initial loading dose of 25 to 30 mg/kg actual body weight should be considered to rapidly achieve goal trough levels that are previously defined. Peak levels are rarely clinically useful, and should not be routinely monitored. Individual doses greater than or equal to 1.5 g should be infused over at least 1.5 to 2 hours.[51] The maximum concentration for any dose should not exceed 5 mg/1 mL.

AMINOGLYCOSIDES

Appropriate dosing of aminoglycosides is imperative to prevent nephrotoxicity and ototoxicity, although these adverse effects can still occur even when goal levels are met, depending on the patient's age, volume status, duration of exposure, and concurrent toxic medications. Any dosing regimen should optimize efficacy while minimizing toxicity. Because aminoglycosides have a long history, they have been widely studied in various patient populations including the obese. There are 2 primary dosing strategies used today: traditional dosing, which involves using lower doses more frequently, or once daily administration, which usually involves nomogram-based higher doses less frequently. Whichever dosing strategy is used, aminoglycosides generally should be dosed based on IBW for patients weighing less than 30% more than their ideal weight. Patients weighing greater than or equal to 30% more than their IBW should be dosed based on their adjusted body weight. (See the section Heparin for formulas). Further dosing adjustments should be made based on the goal peak, trough levels, or random levels depending on the dosing strategy used. Renal and auditory function should be monitored while patients receive aminoglycosides.

SEDATIVES

Although adequate published literature for the recommendation on dosing sedatives is scarce, enough information regarding the pharmacodynamics as well as observed small clinical studies provides some information on certain expectations on the clinical effects of these medications in the obese. Most sedatives, such as propofol, midazolam, and lorazepam, that are used in the critically ill patient are highly lipophilic, so it is assumed that dosing based on actual body weight would be the most appropriate. Although true for propofol and loading doses of benzodiazepines, other important considerations must be noted when using benzodiazepines in the obese patient.

Although many benzodiazepines are dosed based on sedation scales with little regard to weight in a critical care unit, the length of therapy should be taken into account when determining patient requirements or time to awaken in an obese patient. Some small pharmacokinetic studies have demonstrated that the Vd is significantly elevated in obese patients when compared with nonobese controls, which in turn has led to significant elevations in elimination half-life. As a result, lorazepam, midazolam, and diazepam dose requirements can be expected to decrease over time with continuous infusions. Furthermore, because of the longer half-lives in obese patients, the time to awaken can become unpredictable and prolonged after just 48 hours of continuous infusion in the obese critically ill patient. Accurate neurologic examinations and assessments may be obtained only after appropriate time has been given in the obese patient after drug cessation, which is usually much longer then the published kinetic literature. The half-lives of these agents may be tripled or quadrupled in some obese patients when compared with nonobese controls.[52]

Unlike the benzodiazepines, propofol may be dosed based on actual body weight in the obese critically ill patient when used as a continuous infusion. The kinetics (Vd and half-life) of propofol remains very predictable and unchanged in the obese patient.[52]

SUMMARY

Despite the growing epidemic of obesity in the United States, dosing medications in such patients remains poorly studied and understood. Most recommendations are based on small independent studies, case reports, and expert opinion. Applying manufacturer kinetics and dosing recommendations in the obese patient may result in toxicity or treatment failure, leading to increased morbidity, mortality, and hospital length of stay.

REFERENCES

1. Cheymol G. Clinical pharmacokinetics of drugs in obesity: an update. Clin Pharm 1993;25:103–14.
2. Salazar DE, Corcoran GB. Predicting creatinine clearance and renal drug clearance in obese patients from estimated fat-free body mass. Am J Med 1988;84:1053–60.
3. Stockholm KH, Brochner-Mortensen J, Hoilund-Carlson PF. Increased glomerular filtration rate and adrenocortical function in obese women. Int J Obes 1980;4:57–63.
4. Abernethy DR, Greenblatt DJ. Pharmacokinetics of drugs in obesity. Clin Pharm 1982;7:108–24.
5. Blouin RA, Kolpek JH, Man HJ. Influence of obesity on drug disposition. Clin Pharm 1987;6:706–14.
6. Weant KA, Armistead JA, Ladha AM, et al. Cost effectiveness of a clinical pharmacist on a neurosurgical team. Neurosurgery 2009;65(5):946–50.
7. MacLaren R, Bond CA. Effects of pharmacist participation in intensive care units on clinical and economic outcomes of critically ill patients with thromboembolic or infarction-related events. Pharmacotherapy 2009;29(7):761–8.
8. Montazeri M, Cook D. Impact of a clinical pharmacist in a multidisciplinary intensive care unit. Crit Care Med 1994;22(6):1044–8.
9. MacLaren R, Bond C, Martin S, et al. Clinical and economic outcomes of involving pharmacists in the direct care of critically ill patients with infections. Crit Care Med 2008;36(12):3184–9.
10. Rondina MT, Wheeler M, Rodgers GM, et al. Weight-based dosing of enoxaparin for VTE prophylaxis in morbidly obese, medically-ill patients. Thromb Res 2010;125(3):220–3.
11. Davidson BL, Büller HR, Decousus H, et al. Effect of obesity on outcomes after fondaparinux, enoxaparin, or heparin treatment for acute venous thromboembolism in the Matisse trials. J Thromb Haemostasis 2007;5:1191–4.

12. Clark NP. Low-molecular-weight heparin use in the obese, elderly, and in renal insufficiency. Thromb Res 2008;123:S58–61.
13. Barba R, Marco J, Martín-Alvarez H, et al. The influence of extreme body weight on clinical outcome of patients with venous thromboembolism: findings from a prospective registry (RIETE). J Thromb Haemost 2005;3:856–62.
14. Hirsh J, Bauer KA, Donati MB, et al. Parenteral anticoagulants: American College of Chest Physicians Evidence-Based Clinical Practice Guidelines (8th edition). Chest 2008;133(6):141S–59S.
15. Rowan B, Kuhl D, Lee M, et al. Anti-Xa levels in bariatric surgery patients receiving prophylactic enoxaparin. Obes Surg 2008;18:162–6.
16. Borkgren-Okonek M, Hart R, Pantano J, et al. Enoxaparin thromboprophylaxis in gastric bypass patients: extended duration, dose stratification, and antifactor Xa activity. Surg Obes Relat Dis 2008;4:625–31.
17. Simone E, Madan A, Tichansky D, et al. Comparison of two low-molecular-weight heparin dosing regimens for patients undergoing laparoscopic bariatric surgery. Surg Endosc 2008;22:2392–5.
18. Raschke RA, Reilly BM, Guidry JR, et al. The weight-based heparin dosing nomogram compared with a standard care nomogram. Ann Intern Med 1993;119:874.
19. Hull RD, Raskob GE, Rosenbloom D, et al. Optimal therapeutic level of heparin therapy in patients with venous thrombosis. Arch Intern Med 1992;152:1589–95.
20. Hull RD, Raskob GE, Hirsh J, et al. Continuous intravenous heparin compared with intermittent subcutaneous heparin in the initial treatment of proximal-vein thrombosis. N Engl J Med 1986;315:1109–14.
21. Spruill WJ, Wade WE, Huckaby G, et al. Achievement of anticoagulation by using weight based heparin dosing protocol for obese and non-obese patients. Am J Health Syst Pharm 2001;15:2143–6.
22. Ellison MJ, Sawyer WT, Mills TC. Calculation of heparin dosage in a morbidly obese woman. Clin Pharm 1989;8:65–8.
23. Yee WP, Norton LL. Optimal weight base for a weight-based heparin dosing protocol. Am J Health Syst Pharm 1998;55:159–62.
24. Schwiesow S, Wessell A, Steyer T. Use of a modified dosing weight for heparin therapy in a morbidly obese patient. Ann Pharmacother 2005;39:753–6.
25. Bauer S, Ou N, Dreesman B, et al. Effect of body mass index on bleeding frequency and activated partial thromboplastin time in weight based dosing of unfractionated heparin: a retrospective cohort study. Mayo Clin Proc 2009; 84(12):1073–8.
26. Anand SS, Yusuf S, Pogue J, et al. Relationship of activated partial thromboplastin time to coronary events and bleeding in patients with acute coronary syndromes who receive heparin. Circulation 2003;107:2884–8.
27. Myzienski A, Lutz M, Smythe M. Unfractionated heparin dosing for venous thromboembolism in morbidly obese patients: case report and review of the literature. Pharmacotherapy 2010;30(3):105e–12e.
28. Miller MT, Rovito P. An approach to venous thromboembolism prophylaxis in laparoscopic roux-en-y gastric bypass surgery. Obes Surg 2004;14:731–7.
29. Geerts W, Bergqvist D, Pineo G, et al. Prevention of venous thromboembolism American College of Chest Physicians Evidence-Based Clinical Practice Guidelines (8th edition). Chest 2008;133(6):381S–453S.
30. Bernard GR, Vincent JL, Laterre PF, et al. Efficacy and safety of recombinant human activated protein C for severe sepsis. N Engl J Med 2001;344:699–709.
31. Levy H, Small D, Heiselman D, et al. Obesity does not alter the pharmacokinetics of drotrecogin alfa (activated) in severe sepsis. Ann Pharmacother 2005;39:262–7.

32. Argatroban [package insert]. Research triangle park, NC: GlaxoSmithKline; 2005.
33. Cox DS, Kleiman NS, Boyle DA, et al. Pharmacokinetics and pharmacodynamics of argatroban in combination with a platelet glycoprotein IIb/IIIa receptor antagonist in patients undergoing percutaneous coronary intervention. J Clin Pharmacol 2004;44:981–90.
34. Hursting M, Jang I. Effect of body mass index on argatroban therapy during percutaneous coronary intervention. J Thromb Thrombolysis 2008;25:273–9.
35. Rice L, Hursting M, Baillie M, et al. Argatroban anticoagulation in obese versus nonobese patients: implications for treating heparin-induced thrombocytopenia. J Clin Pharmacol 2007;47:1028–34.
36. Keegan S, Gallagher E, Ernst N, et al. Effects of critical illness and organ failure on therapeutic argatroban dosage requirements in patients with suspected confirmed heparin-induced thrombocytopenia. Ann Pharmacother 2009;43(1):19–27.
37. Peck CC, Cross JT. "Getting the dose right": facts a blueprint and encouragements. Clin Pharmacol Ther 2007;82:2–14.
38. Yost RL, Deredorf H. Disposition of cefotaxime and its desacetyl metabolite in morbidly obese male and female subjects. Ther Drug Monit 1986;8:189–94.
39. Forse RA, Karam B, Burlingham BT, et al. Antibiotic prophylaxis for surgery in morbidly obese patients. Surgery 1989;106:750–7.
40. Manjunath PP, Bearden DT. Antimicrobial dosing consideration in obese patients. Pharmacotherapy 2007;27(8):1081–91.
41. Newman D, Scheetz MH, Oluwadamilola AA, et al. Serum piperacillin/tazobactam pharmacokinetics in a morbidly obese individual. Ann Pharmacother 2007;41:1734–9.
42. Tam VH, McKinnon PS, Akins RL, et al. Pharmacodynamics of cefepime in patients with gram-negative infections. J Antimicrob Chemother 2002;50:425–8.
43. Chen M, Nafziger AN, Drusano GL, et al. Comparative pharmacokinetics and pharmacodynamic target attainment of ertapenem in normal-weight, obese, and extremely obese adults. Antimicrob Agents Chemother 2006;50(4):1222–7.
44. Stein GE, Schooley SL, Peloquim CA, et al. Pharmacokinetics and pharmacodynamics of linezolid in obese patients with cellulitis. Ann Pharmacother 2005;39:427–32.
45. Andes D, van Ogtrop ML, Peng J, et al. In vivo pharmacodynamics of a new oxazolidinone (linezolid). Antimicrob Agents Chemother 2002;46:3484–9.
46. Dvorchik BH, Damphousse D. The pharmacokinetics of daptomycin in moderately obese, morbidly obese and matched nonobese subjects. J Clin Pharmacol 2005;45:48–56.
47. Tedesco KL, Rybak MJ. Daptomycin. Pharmacotherapy 2004;24:41–57.
48. Manjunath PP, Norenberg TA, Anderson T, et al. Influence of morbid obesity on the single-dose pharmacokinetics of daptomycin. Antimicrob Agents Chemother 2007;51(8):2741–7.
49. Allard S, Kinzig M, Boivin G, et al. Intravenous ciprofloxacin disposition in obesity. Clin Pharmacol Ther 1993;53:368–73.
50. Caldwell JB. Intravenous ciprofloxacin dosing in morbidly obese patient. Ann Pharmacother 1994;28:806.
51. Rybak M, Lomaestro B, Rotschafer J, et al. Therapeutic monitoring of vancomycin in adult patients: a consensus review of the American Society Health-System pharmacists, the Infectious Diseases Society of America, and the Society of Infectious Diseases Pharmacists. Am J Health Syst Pharm 2009;66:82–98.
52. Casati A, Putzu M. Anesthesia in the obese patient: pharmacokinetic considerations. J Clin Anesth 2005;17:134–45.

Trauma in Obese Patients

Christine C. Toevs, MD, FCCM

KEYWORDS

- Bariatric trauma • Obesity and seat belts
- Obesity and damage control surgery
- Obesity and trauma in pediatric population
- Obesity and burns

As the American population grows larger in terms of weight and body mass index (BMI) each year, a greater percentage of patients admitted to the trauma service are overweight or obese. Obese patients do not have the same injury patterns or outcomes of normal-weight patients. This article reviews some of the latest data regarding the injury patterns, outcomes, and areas of further studies in the obese trauma population.

OBESITY AND SEAT BELT USE

One of the factors contributing to a 50% reduction of motor vehicle crash-related injuries and deaths is seat belt use. One recent study documenting the use of seat belts in obesity is from Vanderbilt in Nashville, Tennessee.[1] Schlundt and colleagues retrospectively investigated the association between BMI and seat belt usage using the 2002 Behavioral Risk Factor Surveillance System survey. Their data show that seat belt use decreases linearly with increasing BMI. A total of 82.6% of individuals with a BMI less than or equal to 24.9 used a seat belt versus 69.8% of individuals with a BMI greater than or equal to 40.0. The investigators concluded that American motorists are unnecessarily at risk for death or injury in motor vehicle crashes (MVCs) because of obesity.

Zarzaur and Marshall[2] at Memphis, Tennessee investigated the injury patterns of seat belt use in obese and nonobese patients. Using the National Automotive Sampling System Crashworthiness Data System, data for 9313 occupants were available. Comparing obese and nonobese occupants with and without seat belts, the investigators determined that no seat belt use increased the odds of death in intra-abdominal injury in obese occupants. For those obese occupants who wore seat belts, neither mortality nor intra-abdominal injury were increased compared with belted nonobese occupants.

The author has nothing to disclose.
Roanoke, VA, USA
E-mail address: ctoevs@aol.com

The risk for intra-abdominal injury in obesity was evaluated by Arbabi and colleagues[3] at the University of Michigan. He and his colleagues specifically queried their trauma database to determine if there was a cushion effect of obesity in MVCs. The investigators noted that obesity did provide an increase in insulating tissue that seemed to protect against intra-abdominal injury. However, the severity of lower-extremity injuries increased with increasing BMI. They did not specifically address seat belt use but rather looked at size as a determinant of injury.

OBESITY AND INJURY RISK IN CHILDREN

Safety of children in motor vehicles has been a major public safety issue for years as demonstrated by the use of car seats and not allowing children in the front seat. Pollack and colleagues[4] investigated the risk for injury specifically in overweight and obese children. They used data from the Partners for Child Passenger Safety study using crash data. They demonstrated a larger percentage of injuries to overweight and obese children (34% of children). Pollack concluded obesity in children in MVCs was a risk for upper-extremity and lower-extremity injuries.

Haricharan and colleagues[5] followed up with another study investigating the injury patterns among obese children in MVCs. In children aged 2 to 5 years, obesity increased the risk for severe head and thoracic injuries. In children aged 6 to 13 years, obesity increased the risk for severe thoracic and lower-extremity injuries. As the children aged, their injury patterns became more like adults, with 14- to17-year old children having an increased risk for lower-extremity injuries and a decreased risk for abdominal and head injuries.

Rana and colleagues,[6] in a retrospective review of the pediatric trauma population at the Children's Hospital in Columbus, Ohio, also found an increased incidence of extremity fractures in obese children. This study did note a decreased incidence of closed head injury and intra-abdominal injuries in obese children. This study also demonstrated an increased risk for decubitus ulcer and venous thromboembolism (VTE) in obese children, paralleling the data in obese adults.

OBESITY AND FRACTURES

To further evaluate the role of obesity in pelvis fractures, Bansal and colleagues[7] queried the Crash Injury Research and Engineering Network. The investigators evaluated 244 occupants with nearside impacts who sustained pelvic fractures. Obese and overweight occupants were less likely to have a pelvis fracture compared with normal-weight occupants. Their study concluded that obesity offers a protective subcutaneous layer of fat over the pelvis. Occupants with a higher BMI and pelvis fracture have more severe injuries overall, which may be caused by their larger size increasing the likelihood of direct compression.

Maheshwari and colleagues[8] evaluated outcomes of subjects with femur and tibia fractures at their Level 1 trauma center in Seattle, Washington. Of 665 subjects (31% obese) there was no difference in mortality between obese subjects and normal-weight subjects. The obese subjects had more severe injury patterns in the distal femur fracture. There were no differences (at baseline or at 6 and 12 months after injury) between the groups using the 36-Item Short Form Health Survey instrument.

OBESITY AND OUTCOMES

Newell and colleagues[9] investigated the risk for increased BMI on morbidity and mortality in critically injured subjects with blunt trauma. A total of 1543 subjects with blunt trauma from 2001 to 2005 were identified in their Level 1 trauma registry. The investigators found that obesity was not a risk for increased mortality. However, obesity did increase the risk for hospital and ICU length of stay, ventilator support, acute respiratory distress syndrome (ARDS), pneumonia, and acute respiratory failure. The investigators attributed the increase in pulmonary complications in obese subjects to underlying respiratory disorders, such as chronic obstructive pulmonary disease, sleep apnea, and obesity hypoventilation syndrome. They also demonstrated increasing complications (organ dysfunction, VTE, and decubitus ulcer formation) in obese subjects critically injured after blunt trauma.

The risk for obesity extends to burn patients. Carpenter and colleagues[10] at the Burn Center at Washington Hospital Center noted that obese subjects with burn injuries were 4.1 times more likely to have length of stay greater than or equal to 7 days. They also noted a 2.6-fold increase in mortality in obese subjects with burn injuries.

Farrell and colleagues[11] at Loyola investigated the functional outcome of obese patients with burn injuries. Obese subjects, regardless of burn size, had lower functional independence measure scores. Elderly subjects who were obese were less likely to be discharged home even with less severe burns. The investigators concluded by stating their study supports the data of obesity contributing to functional decline in older patients.

OBESITY AND DAMAGE CONTROL SURGERY

Damage control surgery is now considered routine in the management of complex trauma patients with acidosis, coagulopathy, and hypothermia. University of Alabama investigated the outcomes of obese patients with damage control laparotomy.[12] Haricharan reviewed data from 48 normal-weight subjects, 54 overweight subjects, and 46 obese subjects. Although there was no difference in mortality between the groups, the subjects with a normal BMI had a shorter time to complete closure of the abdomen than the overweight or obese groups. The obese group had an increased risk for sepsis. The investigators concluded that BMI has a significant impact on time to definitive closure of the abdomen.

Duchesne and colleagues[13] also investigated the impact of obesity in 104 subjects receiving damage control laparotomy. The obese subjects were more likely to develop postoperative infectious complications, multisystem organ failure, and mortality after damage control laparotomy. They did not note a difference in ARDS in this subject population.

OBESITY AND TRAUMATIC BRAIN INJURY

Brown and colleagues[14] queried their Level 1 trauma database in Los Angeles to evaluate the relationship between BMI and traumatic brain injury (TBI). A total of 129 of 690 subjects with TBI were obese and admitted to the ICU. Obese patients with a TBI had a higher mortality (36% vs 25%). Stepwise logistic regression did not identify obesity as in independent risk factor for morbidity or mortality in their subject population.

Tagliaferri and colleagues[15] used the National Automotive Sampling System Database to analyze data regarding obesity and traumatic brain injury. They evaluated 5918 subjects from this database and concluded obesity increased the risk for mortality and injury severity. Obesity also increased the risk for traumatic brain injury. Although this study differs from other studies that do not show an increase in TBI, they state that many other studies exclude subjects who die in the first 24 hours, of which a high proportion have TBI.

OBESITY AND GENOMICS IN TRAUMA

To further delineate the role of obesity in outcomes in patients who are critically injured, several studies have begun to investigate the role of genes and inflammatory response. Collier and colleagues[16] at Vanderbilt investigated visceral adiposity and inflammatory markers. They compared 140 subjects with visceral adiposity to 141 subjects with subcutaneous adiposity as determined by CT scan. They took one blood sample at 48 hours after injury for cytokine levels (IL-1, 2, 4, 6, 8, 10 and tumor necrosis factor). There was no statistical difference between the two groups in cytokine levels. They concluded that the acute inflammatory response of severe injury likely overwhelms the subclinical inflammation associated with obesity in the chronic setting.

Winfield and colleagues,[17] at University of Florida, Gainesville, used microarray data to evaluate differences in inflammatory responses in injured obese and nonobese subjects. They did not note a difference between the two groups, but did determine that base deficit is slower to return to normal in obese patients and may contribute to the mortality and late genomic variation seen in patients with increased BMI. They also state that the resolution of the inflammatory response may vary between obese and nonobese patients, but more data are needed to delineate this timeline.

SUMMARY

Overweight and obese patients who are traumatically injured have different injury patterns than normal-weight patients. Obese patients are more likely to have extremity fractures and potentially TBIs and less likely to have intra-abdominal injuries. Should damage control laparotomy be required, obese patients take longer to reach complete closure of the abdomen and have higher sepsis-related complications. Obese children also follow the same injury patterns, especially as they reach adulthood. Some of these injury patterns appear to be related to decreased seat belt use and cushioning of intra-abdominal contents by visceral fat.

Obese patients with burns have poorer functional outcomes, longer length of stay, and higher mortality. Obese patients overall are more likely to have VTE, decubitus, and sepsis-related complications. Obesity also appears to affect resuscitation and time to normalization of base deficit. The data on mortality are mixed and appear to be related to determination of exclusion criteria. Studies are currently underway to evaluate the role of genomics in the outcomes of obese trauma patients.

REFERENCES

1. Schlundt DG, Briggs NC, Miller ST, et al. BMI and seatbelt use. Obesity (Silver Spring) 2007;15(11):2541–5.
2. Zarzaur BL, Marshall SW. Motor vehicle crashes obesity and seat belt use: a deadly combination? J Trauma 2008;64(2):412–9.
3. Arbabi S, Wahl WL, Hemmila MR, et al. The cushion effect. J Trauma 2003;54(6): 1090–3.
4. Pollack KM, Xie D, Arbogast KB, et al. Body mass index and injury risk among US children 9–15 years old in motor vehicle crashes. Inj Prev 2008;14(6):366–71.
5. Haricharan RN, Griffin RL, Barnhart DC, et al. Injury patterns among obese children involved in motor vehicle collisions. J Pediatr Surg 2009;44(6):1218–22.
6. Rana AR, Michalsky MP, Teich S, et al. Childhood obesity: a risk factor for injuries observed at a level-1 trauma center. J Pediatr Surg 2009;44(8):1601–5.

7. Bansal V, Conroy C, Lee J, et al. Is bigger better? The effect of obesity on pelvic fractures after side impact motor vehicle crashes. J Trauma 2009;67(4):709–14.
8. Maheshwari R, Mack CD, Kaufman RP, et al. Severity of injury and outcomes among obese trauma patients with fractures of the femur and tibia: a crash injury research and engineering network study. J Orthop Trauma 2009;23(9):634–9.
9. Newell MA, Bard MR, Goettler CE, et al. Body mass index and outcomes in critically injured blunt trauma patients: weighing the impact. J Am Coll Surg 2007; 204(5):1056–61.
10. Carpenter AM, Hollett LP, Jeng JC, et al. How long a shadow does epidemic obesity cast in the burn unit? A dietitian's analysis of the strengths and weaknesses of the available data in the National Burn Repository. J Burn Care Res 2008;29(1):97–101.
11. Farrell RT, Gamelli RL, Aleem RF, et al. The relationship of body mass index and functional outcomes in patients with acute burns. J Burn Care Res 2008;29(1): 102–8.
12. Haricharan RN, Dooley AC, Weinberg JA, et al. Body mass index affects time to definitive closure after damage control surgery. J Trauma 2009;66(6):1683–7.
13. Duchesne JC, Schmieg RE Jr, Simmons JD, et al. Impact of obesity in damage control laparotomy patients. J Trauma 2009;67(1):108–12.
14. Brown CV, Rhee P, Neville AL, et al. Obesity and traumatic brain injury. J Trauma 2006;61:572–6.
15. Tagliaferri F, Compagnone C, Yoganandan N, et al. Traumatic brain injury after frontal crashes: relationship with body mass index. J Trauma 2009;66(3):727–9.
16. Collier B, Dossett L, Shipman J, et al. Visceral adiposity is not associated with inflammatory markers in trauma patients. J Trauma 2010;68(1):57–61.
17. Winfield RD, Delano MJ, Dixon DJ, et al. Differences in outcome between obese and nonobese patients following severe blunt trauma are not consistent with an early inflammatory genomic response. Crit Care Med 2010;38(1):51–8.

Bariatric Surgery Patients in the ICU

Mary Jane Reed, MD, FCCM, FCCP[a],*, Jon Gabrielsen, MD[b]

KEYWORDS

- Bariatric surgery • Bariatric surgery complications • ICU
- Roux-en-Y gastric bypass

As the incidence of bariatric surgery continues to increase, the medical community should be aware of the most common procedures, resultant anatomy, and possible complications to be better prepared to care for the bariatric surgical patient in all situations.

There are three types of bariatric procedures commonly done. Restrictive procedures have no portion of the absorptive bowel bypassed. Malabsorptive procedures shorten the effective length of a patient's absorptive bowel. Combined procedures have both restrictive and malabsorptive components. Almost all types of commonly done bariatric procedures can be performed either laparoscopically or open.

The most common bariatric procedure in the United States is the Roux-en-Y gastric bypass. It has both restrictive and malapsorptive components. Typically, a 15- to 50-mL gastric pouch is created with a 75- to 200-cm Roux limb connected as an enteroenterostomy to the jejunum, 30- to 50-cm distal to the ligament of Treitz[1,2] (**Fig. 1**).

The biliopancreatic diversion has a partial gastrectomy with dual intestinal limbs forming a common channel distally 50 to 100 cm from the ileocecal valve. One limb made up mostly of duodenum and jejunum drains the biliary tree and pancreatic bed. The second limb is mostly ileum that is connected to the remaining gastric remnant. This allows for more malabsorption leading to weight loss. The duodenal switch is an adaptation of the biliopancreatic diversion, which performs the partial gastrectomy on the greater curvature of the stomach and keeps the pylorus intact[1,3,4] (**Fig. 2**).

The adjustable gastric band is purely restrictive. Usually placed laparoscopically, the band constricts the proximal portion of the stomach, making an approximately 20- to 30-mL pouch. The band has an inner expandable ring that can be adjusted by instilling fluid via a subcutaneous port (using only an approved needle). The

a Departments of General Surgery and Critical Care Medicine, Geisinger Medical Center, Temple University Medical School, 100 North Academy Avenue, Mail Code: 20-37, Danville, PA 17822, USA
b Department of Bariatric Surgery, Geisinger Medical Center, 100 North Academy Avenue, Danville, PA 17822, USA
* Corresponding author.
E-mail address: mreed@geisinger.edu

Crit Care Clin 26 (2010) 695–698
doi:10.1016/j.ccc.2010.09.001
0749-0704/10/$ – see front matter © 2010 Elsevier Inc. All rights reserved.

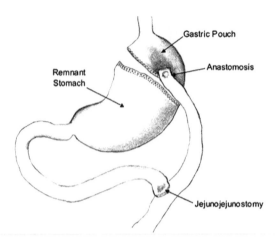

Fig. 1. Vertical banded gastroplasty. (*From* Pandolfino JE, Krishnamoorthy B, Lee TJ. Gastrointestinal complications of obesity surgery. MedGenMed 2004;6. Image reprinted with permission from eMedicine.com, 2010. Available at: http://www.medscape.com/viewarticle/471952. Accessed August 28, 2010.)

band, therefore, can be deflated theoretically in times when more enteral intake is required, such as pregnancy. There is no malabsorption (**Fig. 3**).[1] The second type of purely restrictive procedure is the vertical sleeve gastrectomy, which is now used as a primary bariatric procedure. In this procedure, the partial gastrectomy is done along the greater curvature, leaving the duodenum intact. The resultant pouch holds from 100 to 150 mL.[5]

All bariatric procedures have some operative risk and complications. Where there is division of alimentary tract components and reanastomosis, there is a higher risk of leak, obstruction, or bleeding. Some complications are specific to certain procedures. In Roux-en-Y gastric bypass patients, the gastric remnant can dilate to dangerous

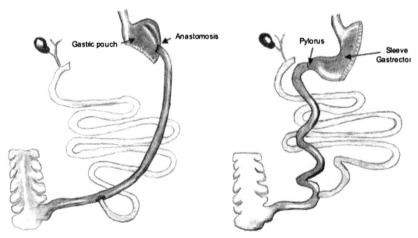

Fig. 2. Adjustable laparoscopic banding. (*From* Pandolfino JE, Krishnamoorthy B, Lee TJ. Gastrointestinal complications of obesity surgery. MedGenMed 2004;6. Image reprinted with permission from eMedicine.com, 2010. Available at: http://www.medscape.com/viewarticle/471952. Accessed August 28, 2010.)

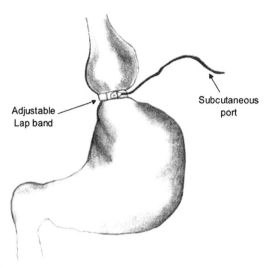

Fig. 3. Roux-en-Y gastric bypass surgery. (*From* Pandolfino JE, Krishnamoorthy B, Lee TJ. Gastrointestinal complications of obesity surgery. MedGenMed 2004;6. Image reprinted with permission from eMedicine.com, 2010. Available at: http://www.medscape.com/viewarticle/471952. Accessed August 28, 2010.)

degrees and present with elevated liver enzymes and signs of sepsis. This dilation cannot be decompressed with nasoenteral tube and may require a gastrostomy tube placed either surgically or with interventional radiology. Because most of the time this gastric remnant dilation is caused by distal intestinal obstruction, it is a surgical condition. Internal hernias are more common in laparoscopic patients than open patients and can cause bowel ischemia and infarction. Prolapse of the stomach through the adjustable gastric band can cause obstruction, which is not relieved with deflation of the band and should be surgically reduced.

Morbidly obese patients often do not exhibit classic signs of peritonitis, such as tenderness to palpation, involuntary guarding, or rebound tenderness. This is thought to be secondary to the increased thickness of the subcutaneous adipose tissue as well as increased thickness of omentum. The signs often seen in morbidly obese patients with peritonitis are tachycardia greater than 120 beats per minute for more than 4 hours, fever, abdominal pain, restlessness, and tenesmus.[1] In addition, bariatric patients will often present with significant shortness of breath as a clinical manifestation of a serious intra-abdominal problem. A recent study of bariatric patients admitted to the ICU with severe post-operative intra-abdominal sepsis and found that the presence of respiratory symptoms led to an incorrect diagnosis in >50% of the patients.[6] When present, these signs are concerning and a bariatric surgeon should be contacted or transfer to a bariatric center should be considered.

Contrast studies, such as CT scan and upper gastrointestinal series, may require slower rate and smaller volumes depending on underlying surgically altered anatomy. If a CT scan is being obtained and the patient can take oral contrast, we have found it helpful in our practice to administer 50–100ml of contrast on the table just prior to scanning (in addition to any other contrast given earlier). This allows contrast to be present in the area of the gastrojejunostomy and pouch at the time of the scan. Additionally, if a CAT scan is being obtained to rule out a pulmonary embolus, it is often wise to administer a small amount of oral contrast on the table and scan the abdomen at the same time since the symptoms of an anastomotic leak may mimic those of pulmonary embolism. Contrast studies do not fully rule out leaks or internal hernias, so in a suspicious clinical setting, emergent surgery may still be required. In patients whose weight prohibits radiographic studies, exploratory surgery may be the first step. Placement of nasogastric tubes or feeding tubes should be reviewed with a bariatric surgeon, especially perioperatively, because they may perforate newly created staple lines.[1]

Cause of bleeding in perioperative bariatric surgery patients can be divided into enteral and intra-abdominal sources. Most bleeding that presents with hematemesis or melena, in the recent post operative patient, is from newly created anastomoses. Bleeding from marginal ulceration of anastomosis can occur weeks to years after initial bariatric operation. Because the clot formation can cause secondary obstruction and possible leak, reoperation is usually performed to control the bleeding. Extraluminal bleeding can be from occult splenic or hepatic injury.

Pressure induced rhabdomyolysis can occur in the postoperative morbidly obese patient. Patients who have prolonged operative time, higher body mass index and diabetes mellitus are at greatest risk.[7] Pain in shoulder, lower legs or buttocks maybe a sign of rhabdomyolysis however often the critical ill patient may not have these complaints. A high index of suspicion of this diagnosis should be maintained.

Because of the malabsorptive portion of most of the bariatric procedures, patients require supplementation. In Roux-en-Y gastric bypass, patients require routine supplementation with iron, calcium, and vitamin B_{12}. More malabsorptive procedures, such as biliopancreatic diversion, require a higher protein diet because more protein is lost.[1] Neurologic abnormalities, such as neuropathies, myopathies, burning feet, and Wernicke-like encephalopathy, have been described in postoperative bariatric surgery patients. Protracted vomiting has been attributed to creating a thiamine deficiency. It is proposed, then, to give thiamine before glucose to any bariatric surgery patient with vomiting.[8]

Fundamental knowledge of altered anatomy and possible complications helps when caring for critically ill obese patients.

REFERENCES

1. Luber S, Fischer D. Care of the bariatric surgery patient in the Emergency Department: bariatric surgery procedures. J Emerg Med 2008;34(1):13–20.
2. Livingston EH. Procedure incidence and in-hospital complication rates of bariatric surgery in the United States. Am J Surg 2004;188:105–10.
3. Scopinaro N. Outcome evaluation after bariatric surgery. Obes Surg 2002;12:253.
4. Scopinaro N, Gianetta E, Adami GF, et al. Biliopancreatic diversion for obesity at eighteen years. Surgery 1996;119:261–8.
5. Pitombo C. Obesity surgery: principles and practice. New York (NY): McGraw Hill Professional; 2008. p.177.
6. Kermarrec N, Marmuse JP, Faivre J, et al. High mortality rate for patients requiring intensive care after surgical revision following bariatric surgery. Obes Surg 2008; 18:171–8.
7. Mognol P, Vignes S, Chosidow D, et al. Rhabmyolysis after laparoscopic bariatric surgery. Obes Surg 2004;14:91–4.
8. Berger JR. The neurological complications of bariatric surgery. Arch Neurol 2004; 61:1185–9.

Special Considerations in the Critically Ill Morbidly Obese Child

Karen Allison Bailey, BSc, MD, FRCSC

KEYWORDS

- Critical care • Morbidly obese • Child • Pediatric
- Special considerations

Obesity has been recognized as an increasing problem not only in North America but globally. With a significant rise in the prevalence of obesity amongst children and adolescents over the past 20 years, the comorbidities associated with obesity are also now emerging at an earlier age. These comorbidities cause specific concern and require special consideration when the morbidly obese child becomes critically ill.

In the United States the prevalence of obesity (body mass index [BMI] >95th percentile) was found to have increased among children aged 2 to 19 years with an age-related prevalence of 12.4% (aged 2–5 years), 17% (aged 6–11 years), and17.6% (aged 12–19 years).[1] The prevalence of children who are overweight (BMI >85th percentile) was found to be 33.3% to 34.1% based on the 2003 to 2006 National Health and Nutrition Examination Survey data.[1] The International Obesity Task Force has estimated that among school-aged children worldwide, as many as 155 million children are overweight or obese.[2]

As with adults, the causes of obesity in children are multiple. Although weight gain is often viewed as simply being caused from taking in more calories than are expended there are many other factors that influence obesity. These factors include heredity, metabolic, behavior, environment, culture, and socioeconomic status. In children, medical conditions and rare syndromes, such as hypothyroidism, Prader-Willi syndrome, and Cushing syndrome, account for a small number of pediatric patients who are morbidly obese but must be considered as potential causes.[3,4]

The rising prevalence of obesity will no doubt cause many pediatric critical care units to face the challenges of managing children who are morbidly obese. Many units are not physically designed to accommodate patients who are morbidly obese and their staff has not been specially trained to care for these patients, which potentially places patients and staff at risk. Weight-appropriate beds, chairs, scales, lifts, and

The author has nothing to disclose.
Pediatric General Surgery, Pediatric Trauma Program, McMaster Children's Hospital, McMaster University, 1200 Main Street West, Room 4E4, Hamilton, ON L8N 3Z5, Canada
E-mail address: kbailey@mcmaster.ca

blood pressure cuffs may not be present to facilitate treatment of morbidly obese patients. Doorways and rooms may be too small to accommodate wider weight-appropriate beds, chairs, lifts, and equipment.

Radiologic imaging can also be problematic in patients who are morbidly obese. The patients' size can limit visualization with all modalities. Increased radiation may be required to adequately penetrate the tissues for plain films. Equipment specifications vary and typically have a maximum of 250 to 450 lb depending on the manufacturer's specifications, which may preclude patients who are morbidly obese from having a CT scan, MRI, or fluoroscopy depending on the equipment available. The gantry size of the CT and MRI scanner, or the space between the table top to the fluoroscopy image intensifier, may also limit the ability to obtain adequate imaging.[5]

The comorbidities associated with morbid obesity have not been extensively studied or reported on specifically in the pediatric critical care population but they need to be carefully considered. Morbid obesity in childhood is clearly associated with increased problems with asthma, obstructive sleep apnea, hypertension, dyslipidemia, impaired glucose tolerance, gastroesophageal reflux, cholelithiasis, osteoarthritis, and liver dysfunction. These complications were once considered to be only long-term effects of obesity that appeared in adulthood, but pediatric studies have shown that they are clearly appearing in childhood.[6,7]

The importance of addressing morbid obesity and the potential for reversing these comorbidities after excess weight is lost has been most clearly demonstrated in the literature in adolescents who have undergone bariatric surgery. Although diet, exercise, and behavioral therapy are essential components in preventing and addressing obesity, sadly they are often inadequate alone. Bariatric surgery, although still considered controversial in children, has been effective in improving and resolving obesity-related comorbidities.[8–10]

Many critically ill children will require ventilatory support so it important to understand that respiratory mechanics may be altered from both a restrictive and obstructive component in patients who are morbidly obese. Chest wall compliance and diaphragmatic excursion may be decreased because of adiposity and its distribution. Atelectasis is a greater problem in the obese population that requires increased diligence to ensure adequate ambulation, pulmonary toilet, and chest physiotherapy as needed.[3,6] Obese children are slower to recover after severe asthma exacerbations and have been found to require longer intensive care unit (ICU) courses and more supplemental oxygen, continuous albuterol, and intravenous steroids in comparison to their lean peers.[11]

As with morbidly obese adults, the airway in morbidly obese pediatric patients may be more difficult to visualize and maintain. Intubation can be more challenging in young patients because of the more anterior position of the airway; this visualization can be further impaired by adiposity. In patients who are morbidly obese, practitioners should be prepared to have assistance readily called for and access to equipment for difficult airway intubation. Training in advanced airway and bronchoscopy skills can be life saving.

Obstructive sleep apnea may require patients to be given continuous positive airway pressure when lethargic or at rest. Some of these morbidly obese children may have had significant issues with night-time oxygen desaturations, which were not detected before hospitalization.[7,12]

Obesity-related hypertension and insulin resistance may lead to significant renal dysfunction, although this usually presents later in life. Morbid obesity may be associated with abnormal liver enzymes; if untreated, it has been associated with nonalcoholic steatohepatitis that can lead to frank liver failure if obesity is not addressed.[13]

Drug doses are often based upon age or weight in children. Some pharmacokinetics are well understood with doses adjusted for renal or hepatic dysfunction in children. In the face of significant excess weight, the resulting changes in pharmacokinetics for children with or without organ dysfunction are not as well defined. As described in the anesthesia literature, when obese pediatric patients receive medications, such as midazolam and fentanyl (which have an increased volume of distribution throughout the body), they are often best administered based upon total body weight. Some medications are distributed to lean tissues predominantly and are better administered to patients according to their ideal body weight.[3,14]

If supplemental enteral or parenteral nutrition is required it is important to consider that patients may require additional medications or liver-protecting strategies because of underlying insulin resistance and hyperlipidemia. Morbid obesity does not equate to adequate nutrition and, if tested, many patients will be found to be deficient in essential nutrients that are needed to promote healing and to fight infection. Although patients are morbidly obese, adequate nutrition is essential to prevent muscle loss. The morbidly obese child may already have difficulty with ambulation and osteoarthritis. Rehabilitation and recovery will be impaired if there is further loss of normal muscle mass caused by inadequate nutrition. Early involvement of physical and occupational therapy should be considered in this patient population.[10]

In the pediatric trauma population, obese children and adolescents appear to have higher complication rates, with longer time on ventilation and longer ICU stays than lean pediatric trauma patients. Specific complications that have been identified as being higher in association with obesity in the pediatric trauma population include wound infection, sepsis, postoperative fistulas, decubitus ulcers, and deep venous thrombosis.[15,16]

The morbidly obese child often appears to be much older than their actual age. Although significantly larger in size than many of their peers, they are not more emotionally mature or able to cope with a critical illness. These patients may be less able to cope with the stresses of a critical illness because depression and psychiatric disease often present hand in hand with morbid obesity. It is important for the critical care team to remember this, so as to compassionately care for their emotional and psychological needs in an age-appropriate manner.[17–19]

A team approach is needed to address all of the special considerations in this patient population. As the severity and prevalence of obesity continues to rise, we must become aware and prepared to treat this patient population. The morbidly obese child is not merely a large child, but a child with many potential complexities and concerns that we must take into account within the critical care setting.

REFERENCES

1. Centers for Disease Control and Prevention. NHANES Surveys (1976–1980 and 2003–2006). Available at: http://www.cdc.gov/obesity/childhood/prevalence.html. Accessed February 15, 2010.
2. International Obesity Task Force. Childhood obesity. Available at: http://www.iotf.org/childhoodobesity.asp. Accessed February 15, 2010.
3. Brenn BR. Anesthesia for pediatric obesity. Anesthesiol Clin North America 2005; 23:745–64.
4. Sharma AJ, Grummer-Strawn LM, Dalenius K, et al. Obesity prevalence among low-income, preschool-aged children-United States, 1998–2008. CDC MMWR Morb Mortal Wkly Rep 2009;58(28):1–2.

5. Inge TH, Lane FD, Vierra M, et al. Managing bariatric patients in a children's hospital: radiologic considerations and limitations. J Pediatr Surg 2005;40(4): 609–17.

6. Kline A. Pediatric obesity in acute and critical care. AACN Adv Crit Care 2008; 19(1):38–46.

7. Noble K. The obesity epidemic: the impact of obesity on the perianesthesia patient. J Perianesth Nurs 2008;23(6):418–25.

8. Inge TH, Xanthakos SA, Zeller MH. Bariatric surgery for pediatric extreme obesity: now or later? Int J Obes (Lond) 2007;31:1–14.

9. Nadler EP, Reddy S, Isenalumhe A, et al. Laparoscopic adjustable gastric banding for morbidly obese adolescents affect android fat loss, resolution of comorbidities and improved metabolic status. J Am Coll Surg 2009;209(5):638–44.

10. Inge TH, Krebs NF, Garcia VF, et al. Bariatric surgery for severely overweight adolescents: concerns and recommendations. Pediatrics 2004;114(1):217–23.

11. Carroll CL, Bhandari A, Zucker AR, et al. Childhood obesity increases duration of therapy during severe asthma exacerbations. Pediatr Crit Care Med 2006;7(6): 527–31.

12. Schwengel DA, Sterni LM, Tunkel DE, et al. Perioperative management of children with obstructive sleep apnea. Anesth Analg 2009;109(1):60–75.

13. Dietz WH. Health consequences of obesity in youth: childhood predictors of adult disease. Pediatrics 1998;101:518–25.

14. Cheymol G. Effects of obesity on pharmacokinetics, implications for drug therapy. Clin Pharmacokinet 2000;39:215–31.

15. Rana AR, Michalsky MP, Teich S, et al. Childhood obesity: a risk factor for injuries observed at a level-1 trauma center. J Polyn Soc 2009;44:1601–5.

16. Brown CVR, Neville AL, Salim A, et al. The impact of obesity on severely injured children and adolescents. J Pediatr Surg 2006;41:88–91.

17. Dixon JB, Dixon ME, O'Brien PE. Depression in association with severe obesity: changes with weight loss. Arch Intern Med 2003;163:2058–65.

18. Mustillo S, Worthman C, Erkanli A, et al. Disorder: developmental trajectories. Pediatrics 2003;111(4):851–9.

19. McIntyre RS, Konarski JZ. Obesity and psychiatric disorders: frequently encountered clinical questions. Focus 2005;3(4):511–9.

Critical Care of the Morbidly Obese in Disaster

James Geiling, MD, FCCM[a,b,]*

KEYWORDS

- Morbidly obese • Obese • Disasters • Critical care
- Emergency management • Special populations

The prevalence of obesity in the United States is increasing, with extreme morbid obesity of body mass index (BMI, calculated as the weight in kilograms divided by height in meters squared) greater than 40 increasing twice as fast as obesity in general. With the increased weight comes an increased risk of comorbidities, including type 2 diabetes mellitus, cardiovascular disease, respiratory problems such as obstructive sleep apnea (OSA) or restrictive lung disease, skin disorders such as intertrigo and cellulitis, and urinary incontinence.[1] Thus, patients exposed to a variety of disasters not only are increasingly overweight but also have an associated number of coexistent medical conditions that require increased support with medical devices and medications.

Recent events support the need to plan for managing these patients. For example, Hurricane Ike in 2008 had a high prevalence of obese patients who strained evacuation and shelter systems. Planning for this patient population is now becoming a requirement for relief organizations, with most considering placing them in special-needs shelters.[2]

Although the focus of this discussion is the effect of disasters on the management of the morbidly obese patient, many formerly obese patients may also have an altered response to the stresses of disasters. Many obese patients who fail to respond to

The author has no financial conflict of interest to disclose.

Funding: There was no funding for this work.

The opinions and assertions contained herein are those of the author and do not necessarily reflect the views or position of the Department of Veterans Affairs or the academic institutions with which the author is affiliated.

a Veterans Affairs Medical Center, 215 North Main Street, White River Junction, VT 05009, USA

b Dartmouth Medical School, New England Center for Emergency Preparedness, One Medical Center Drive Lebanon, NH 03756, USA

* Dartmouth Medical School, New England Center for Emergency Preparedness, One Medical Center Drive Lebanon, NH 03756.

E-mail address: james.geiling@dartmouth.edu

Crit Care Clin 26 (2010) 703–714

doi:10.1016/j.ccc.2010.06.001

0749-0704/10/$ – see front matter. Published by Elsevier Inc.

criticalcare.theclinics.com

changes in lifestyle or medications choose to undergo a variety of bariatric surgical procedures. The most common procedures include gastric banding (which may be adjustable), sleeve gastrectomy, Roux-en-Y gastric bypass, and biliopancreatic diversion with duodenal switch. Some patients treated with these procedures suffer from postoperative gastrointestinal complaints, including nausea, vomiting, the dumping syndrome (especially with the Roux-en-Y procedure), and other complaints such as ulcers, bowel obstructions, hernias, and adhesions.[3] These patients have specific nutritional needs after surgery. Many patients have food intolerances, including intolerance to bread, dairy foods, carbonated beverages, dry or sticky food, or foods of high sugar content. In addition, these patients often require protein-rich foods, and especially in the early postoperative period, they need to avoid dehydration.[4] Thus, the complicated logistics of nutritional support in a disaster may put these patients at risk for a variety of gastrointestinal complaints, poor wound healing, and dehydration. In addition, besides the routine presentation of these complications at the time of a disaster, the signs and symptoms of these adverse effects may also mimic the signs or symptoms of a variety of common disaster-related complications, including blast abdomen, toxin or chemical ingestion, gastrointestinal complications of biologic agents or acute radiation exposure, or simply the overwhelming effects of the stress of experiencing a disaster. Therefore, especially in these patients, a thorough knowledge of the medical and surgical history becomes important in discerning the effects of the previous surgery from that of the acute event.

HOSPITAL IMPACT

The scope of the problem may be greater than anticipated. For example, simply recognizing the problem can be especially difficult, because emergency personnel can accurately predict the weight of patients with a BMI greater than 30 only 23% of the time.[5] Even internal medicine residents who often treat the medical consequences of obesity do not know the BMI required to diagnose obesity 60% of the time; 40% do not even know their own BMI.[6]

Patients presenting to emergency departments during normal daily operations are increasing in number as reflected by national statistics. From 1986 to 2000, patients with a BMI greater than 30 increased from 10% to 20% of the population; those with a BMI greater than 40 increased from 0.5% to 2%. Those with a BMI greater than 50 increased from 1 in 2000 to 1 in 400 persons. More than three-fourths of emergency departments in 2006 reported an increase in the number of these "superobese" patients. These patients require specialized transportation equipment and extra support personnel. Ambulances need special beds, ramps, winches, and other equipments to bring them to the emergency departments. Emergency departments also require expensive equipments such as patient lifters that cost approximately $18,000.[7]

DISASTER CRITICAL CARE

As the patients' weight and mobility requirements increase, so do the resource requirements to meet those needs. Once exposed to a disaster scenario, patients require on-scene treatment and transportation to a facility capable of managing them. Unlike normal events, in which most survivors find their own conveyance to the closest hospital, obese patients will most likely not be able to do that, relying therefore on emergency medical services (EMS). Less critically ill patients may be taken to lower-acuity facilities or, in the setting of a slowly evolving event like pandemic flu, a community surge facility such as an acute care facility. For example, special accommodations may also be needed to get these patients immunized, because it is unlikely that they will be able to get to a community vaccine or medication point of distribution (POD). If hospitalization is required, these patients will need to be managed regionally as is done with pediatric or burn patients at present. Regional Medical Control Centers should monitor what facilities can manage these patients and ensure that proper transportation assets are available to assist in their movement.[8]

In addition, community health planners need to be aware of these patients in their community, in the same way they should be aware of patients with home oxygen or medical devices. If these patients need evacuation because of a pending disaster or sudden event, then the local medical control should be proactive in seeking resources to move them to appropriate care or transportation hubs for moving them out of the region.[9]

When disasters occur, the effect on the health care system depends on the nature of the event. In sudden-impact disasters such as transportation accidents, bombings, or fire, large numbers of patients tend to present to the closest facility over a short time span, typically within 3 hours. The hospital is mostly affected in the emergency department and, perhaps, the operating room. However, more protracted events such as pandemic flu would have a more prolonged effect on intensive care units (ICUs). These valuable resources may quickly become overburdened, requiring resources to surge to meet those needs. Ideally, hospitals discharge less critically ill patients to home, long-term care facilities, or even community disaster centers, leaving staffed ICU beds available for those needing this care. However, because those strategies also become overwhelmed, hospitals will need to expand their internal critical care capabilities with creative approaches to surging equipment, staff, and care space, that is, stuff, staff, and space. Because of the increased needs and comorbidities of obese patients, they pose additional challenges to this surge strategy.[10]

Stuff

Simple measures such as determining vital signs may be challenging in a disaster setting. In a review from France, prehospital management problems of morbidly obese patients included inability to measure blood pressure in 9%, inability to gain venous access in 13%, and difficulty in intubating 20% of the patients, often requiring advanced airways.[11] The routine use of noninvasive blood pressure cuffs may not be useful because of the inherent inaccuracies of the cuff's bladder size to arm circumference.[12] Normal emergency department and ICU procedures may also need additional support, including changed or decreased quality of electrocardiograms, poor radiographic or ultrasonographic imaging, increased reliance on invasive monitoring or procedures, such as diagnostic peritoneal lavage if the patient cannot fit the computed tomographic scanner, and advanced airway support due to oropharynx size or neck mobility limitations.[13]

In 2008, the Task Force on Mass Critical Care reviewed the recommended ventilator characteristics for disaster settings as well as ancillary equipment.[14] Although review of that information reveals no specific recommendations for the needs of the obese patient, it does point to the requirement to ensure the equipment cached for disaster events do, indeed, fit these patients. The ventilator characteristics should meet such patients' needs, although if noninvasive ventilation is considered (which was not recommended by the Task Force), appropriately sized masks must be available. In addition, monitoring equipments such as blood pressure cuffs and pulse oximeters as well as central venous catheters and other tubes and lines must be of sufficient sensitivity and size to care for these patients.

Pharmacologic caches of emergency medications may not always include those that might be most appropriate for this patient population. For example, opioids for pain have a widespread variability in effectiveness with significant interindividual analgesic requirements. Treatment at the higher end of the recommended dosing ranges for a variety of antimicrobials may also be needed. Even corticosteroid use in acute short-term indications may need higher dosing according to adjusted body weight to avoid subtherapeutic effects at lower dosing.[15] Depending on the number and sizes of these patients in the disaster setting, large quantities of medication may be needed to manage this population. As a result of the increased logistic demands, providing enough medications for all patients could be jeopardized.

Obese patients may be on medications to treat their obesity. These medications include sibutramine, phentermine, diethylpropion, orlistat, bupropion, fluoxetine, sertraline, topiramate, and zonisamide. Side effects of these medications, such as tachycardia, increased blood pressure, insomnia, paresthesia, dyspepsia, diarrhea, flatulence, and abdominal pain may mimic or alter normal findings that result from disaster-related trauma or toxin exposure.[16] Also, few, if any, of these medications may be in disaster pharmacology caches, resulting in the risk of acute disruption in their availability for these patients.

Beds can be a challenge, especially in shelter or improvised space. Obese patients often require 2 cots that then need devices to keep the patients safe. Because cots are low to the ground, getting the patient on and out of the bed can be difficult for the staff. In addition, these cots tend to lie flat; obese patients often have comorbidities such as congestive heart failure or especially OSA that necessitate an upright position in bed. They have also been noted to have difficulty in clearing secretions when recumbent.[17] Also, in shelters, observed snoring and OSA in patients have prompted urgent "disaster sleep studies" and have been shown to adversely affect others in the shelter, disturbing their sleep.[18] Shelters also have limited toilet and bathing facilities. Obese patients may require special accommodations for these routine functions. For example, nurses are often not aware of the weight limitations of toilets or bedside commode, leading to potential patient safety challenges.[19]

The US Department of Health and Human Services has developed and continues to improve several fully equipped Federal Medical Stations (FMS) that can deploy to disaster locations. The FMS provide a 250-bed capability that includes 3 days of medical supplies, equipment, and pharmaceuticals. FMS are deployed to disaster locations and set up in buildings of convenience, such as convention centers, arenas, or warehouses. Although normally configured to manage low-acuity patients, they can also, with additional resources, support more critically ill patients. The FMS that were established in 2008 after the Hurricanes Gustav and Ike had approximately 20% of their critical patients classified as morbidly obese (Yeskey K, Deputy Assistant Secretary, Director, Office of Preparedness and Emergency Operations, Assistant Secretary for Preparedness and Response, Department of Health and Human Services, personal communication, February 18, 2010), and this diagnosis, which did not exist previously, has been added to electronic health records for patients. As part of the special-needs configuration of FMS, a bariatric set comprising 5 special electric beds and other bariatric items has been prepared. Special equipments in these sets include:

1. Electric beds with 270-kg capacity
2. Portable commodes with 450-kg capacity
3. Continuous positive airway pressure (CPAP) machines
4. CPAP masks
5. Obesity gowns
6. Patient hydraulic lifts with 450-kg capacity
7. Transfer bench with 315-kg capacity

8. Walkers with 315-kg capacity
9. Wheelchairs with 315-kg capacity.

(Donohue J, Emergency Management Specialist/FMS Division Strategic National Stockpile, Office of Public Health Preparedness and Response (OPHPR) Centers for Disease Control and Prevention, personal communication, February 18, 2010).

Staff

Paramount in managing morbidly obese patients is the safety of the staff. During normal operations, many health care facilities as well as first-responder or transportation assets lack appropriate weight-based assistance devices. Even if available, these patients require increased number of staff to help safely move them.[20] In disaster settings where medical staff may have limited availability and security, EMS, volunteers, and other nonmedical personnel may be used to assist health care workers in patient movement, lifting, and other physical tasks.[17]

In addition to the increased number of staff required to manage obese patients, the staff themselves are similarly increasing in size along with the general population, putting themselves at risk for injuries and illnesses related to their size. EMS personnel are especially at risk because of the physical demands placed on them, especially in disaster settings. Of almost 400 consecutive fire and ambulance recruits in Massachusetts, all staff had a BMI greater than 25, with 33% having a BMI greater than 30.[21]

Space

The Task Force on Mass Critical Care recommends that in disaster settings, critical care occurs in hospitals and not in field hospitals or contingency facilities in the community because of the special needs of critically ill patients, such as hospital beds, infection-control barriers, specialized equipments (eg, ventilators), oxygen, and other needs.[14] These needs are especially relevant to the obese patient. However, the repurposing of surge space in a hospital, such as postanesthesia care units, intermediate care units, endoscopy suites, and surgicenters, implies that those spaces have the stuff and staff to manage the patients. As hospitals develop their own mechanisms for managing obese patients, the locations and equipment to manage them, such as patient lifts, may not be universally available in these surge spaces, thereby necessarily accommodating these patients in the few areas already designated for their needs.

Transportation

Clearly, the morbidly obese patient requires additional or special transportation assets. At home or care facility, large chairs, litters or stretchers, evacuation devices or sleds, or other transport devices must be available. Movement to the ambulance requires special transport stretchers, which need to accommodate a variety of patient positions. Even loading the patient on to the vehicle may require special ramps or winches.[22] This special equipment is expensive and the additional manpower and time needed to move these patients can be significant. For example, 22 firefighters and EMS personnel reportedly took 2.5 hours to move a woman weighing 347.4 kg out of the narrow doorway of her town house to the ambulance.[7]

External resources including ground and air vehicles all have specific weight and load restrictions, some of which may further affect movement depending on weather conditions. Bulky and heavier patients put additional strains on vehicles and even require more fuel to carry the increased load. In addition, just because of their size, additional equipments, and extra support persons there is less room for nonobese patients; thereby increasing the evacuation needs, such as more vehicles, aircraft sorties, and so on.

Normal evacuation procedures also need to be altered with innovative solutions. A patient weighing 495 kg required transfer from a rural community hospital to a tertiary care facility for an apparent acute abdomen. Because normal vehicle and transport devices had only 382.5-kg capacity, the community provider solicited the help of the state's national guard. The patient was then transferred in his bed to the large CH-47 Chinook helicopter, the US Army's tandem-rotor heavy-lift helicopter for transport, along with hospital support personnel.[23] Because of the urgency, a local paramedic unit that was not trained in aeromedical evacuation procedures provided support in the air. On arrival at the receiving facility, the downdraft of the helicopter resulted in receiving personnel being blown about the landing area and local damage to nearby cars (Hinds J, Operations Manager, Dartmouth-Hitchcock Advanced Response Team, personal communication, January 7, 2010). Although the result was a successful patient transfer, the scenario highlights the high resource demands these patients would place on an EMS system when, in a disaster, resources would be severely constrained.

Ideally, emergency medical plans would include vehicles capable of managing these patients. They should be comfortable for the patient, accommodate the increased support persons needed, and ease patient movement without causing lifting injuries. However, the challenge is that such a resource would be expensive to purchase and maintain; expensive to equip, staff, and train; and is in short supply.

Given the requirements and restrictions in moving obese patients, pressure-induced rhabdomyolysis may occur. Although rare, it is a well-described complication of bariatric surgery, and thus the complication could occur not only in the operating room but also under similar circumstances in which patients are immobile for prolonged periods during transport.[24] Acute compartment syndrome may also develop as a consequence and is difficult to diagnose in already compromised extremities or if patients are sedated and cannot provide adequate history of pain.

MANAGEMENT OF OBESE PATIENTS IN SPECIFIC DISASTERS
Trauma, Blast, and Burn Injury

Traumatic injury is often the consequence of disasters and its effect on the morbidly obese patient must be considered in planning support to these patients. Once hospitalized, severely obese patients with a BMI greater than 30 have higher mortality than obese patients. Increased injury severity score and BMI are independent determinants of outcome with obese patients having increased pulmonary, renal, and thromboembolic complications.[25] Obese patients who survive also require longer periods of mechanical ventilation and hospitalization.[26] However, the mortality data on these patients suffering blunt traumatic injury are not consistent.[27] In fact, although obese patients may have longer hospitalizations, which must be considered in planning health care system capabilities, they do not seem to suffer increased ICU or hospital mortality, which may actually be lower.[28]

Most assume that airway management in trauma patients is compromised by the physical changes and limitations in the morbidly obese. However, data demonstrating this problem are limited. In comparison with lean and overweight patients, a review of airway management experience at a level 1 trauma facility showed no difference in difficult intubations. However, an important caveat is that 92% of the intubations were conducted by an experienced anesthesia team, with 6% by experienced emergency department personnel. In short, although classically these patients are thought to have challenging airway management issues, in experienced hands this has not been demonstrated.[29]

Blast injuries result in primary (such as tympanic membrane rupture), secondary (from blast projectiles), tertiary (from being projected into an obstacle), and quaternary (from associated injuries such as burns) injuries. Prognostic factors include the magnitude of the explosion, building collapse, time interval to treatment, triage accuracy, and immediacy of medical or surgical support.[30] Several of these prognostic factors may be affected by the size of the patient, including accuracy of the triage, ability to transport the patient, and the resources needed to get the patient immediately to the operating room. Specific effects of the blast may also be affected by the size of the patient, including the development of intestinal injuries. The potential cushioning effect of a pannus could serve as a protective barrier, yet diagnosis of acute blast abdomen may be challenging depending on ultrasonography or computerized axial tomographic scan capabilities; peritoneal lavage may need to be performed. Large wounds in patients with significant subcutaneous tissue involvement may be predisposed to poor wound healing.

Burn management in these patients should follow normal protocols. But again, the challenges lie in the details. Clearly, with increased body surface area these patients are at risk for more injury and hence higher fluid requirements and infection risk. Obesity itself predisposes these patients to increased morbidity (ie, infection), ventilatory support, insulin requirements, antibiotic usage, and perhaps immunologic markers.[31] Skin grafting could be potentially problematic, particularly because these patients may already be at risk for decubitus stasis changes. Ideally, these patients would be managed in a burn center, thereby highlighting the transportation challenges discussed earlier.

Natural Disasters and Mass Casualty Crush Syndrome

Natural disasters have distinct injury patterns associated with the type of disaster. The greatest challenge early in natural disasters is to determine the extent of damage and hence the number of casualties. Initial impressions and estimates, on which health care decisions are made, are often inaccurate. As a result, secondary disasters from misallocation of resources often develop. Clearly, the type of disaster and especially its geopolitical location determine the effect of obese patients on the response effort. For example, in the immediate aftermath of the Haiti earthquake of 2010, there were no obese patients in the native population and hence management of these patients was not an issue. Obesity in the responders, however, did pose challenges, because many of the responsders were not acclimated to the heat or physical demands of the event (Geiling J, personal observation, 2010).

Many natural disasters result in large numbers of crush injuries. Clearly, obese persons are at an increased risk of being exposed because of their baseline-limited mobility. Extraction of these patients poses significant challenges as a result of the increased body surface area being trapped and additional equipment and personnel needed to conduct the extraction. Once trapped, their limbs of increased mass, even if mostly adipose tissue, pose a risk for development of crush injury with the resultant rhabdomyolysis and acute kidney injury.[32] Compartment syndrome in injured extremities may also develop, especially as patients are extracted and hydrated. The classic findings of pulselessness, pallor, absence of pain, poikilothermia, and paralysis may be difficult to obese extremities, putting additional risk to injured extremities.

Chemical, Biologic, and Radiologic Disasters

Chemical disasters, not caused by industrial or transportational accidents, result from the use of nerve agents, vesicants, cyanides, pulmonary agents, and riot-control or other nonlethal agents. Primary to the management of these patients is to remove them from the contaminated environment and decontaminate them. The challenge of moving these patients as has been discussed in other settings puts them at risk of additional or prolonged exposures. Decontamination can be either dry (mostly accomplished by removing a survivor's clothes) or wet (by having patients washed off with soap and water). Ambulatory patients can do this themselves, but nonambulatory patients require assistance. Again, given their movement constraints, additional support personnel and special equipment must be available to not only decontaminate these special patients but also initiate treatment.

Care for most chemical casualties is supportive airway, breathing with mechanical ventilation if needed, intravenous fluids, and so forth. The challenges in providing this care for obese patients have already been discussed. Several agents have specific antidotes, including atropine and pralidoxime for nerve agents and amyl or sodium nitrite with sodium thiosulfate or hydroxocobalamin for cyanide poisoning.[33] All of these agents have standard recommended dosing that is not weight based. However, for example, if atropine is recommended to be used in 2-mg intervals until secretions caused by nerve agents decrease, large volumes of medications may be needed to manage these patients.

Biologic disasters result from either the intentional release of a bioweapon or, more likely, a naturally occurring event, such as the outbreak of severe acute respiratory syndrome (SARS) in 2003 or H1N1 in 2009. Management of obese patients in these settings poses no specific change in care other than the challenges faced in the routine outpatient and inpatient or ICU care already discussed. Community response efforts to an outbreak may require isolation or quarantine. Such an intervention by public health authorities would further distance these patients from the care and support they normally require from community resources. Depending on their mobility, they may be unable to attend POD centers that may be established to distribute medications or immunizations, thereby putting them at increased risk of contracting the disease at hand.

Once ill and hospitalized, several classic agents require isolation precautions to minimize spread of the contagion. Smallpox, viral hemorrhagic fevers, and H1N1 or other novel influenzas require airborne and contact precautions, whereas plague and SARS require droplet and contact precautions. Thus, management of the obese patients in these settings requires additional resources not normally needed for normal patients in ICU. For example, the simple act of moving these patients or responding to ventilator alarms or other emergencies requires more personnel, with additional personal protective equipment and supplies. Such gear will already likely be in short supply, thereby already aggravating the shortage.[34]

Radiation disasters can take several forms: a bomb and low levels of radiation that is contaminant purposely implanted to create widespread contamination (through a radiation dispersal device, also known as a dirty bomb), an accidental or intentional release of radiation from a nuclear power plant or processing center, or a nuclear fission device or atomic bomb. In short, bombs or explosions associated with radiation require patient decontamination with removal of clothing and washing the body and acute management of traumatic injuries. The challenges of managing obese patients during decontamination and trauma management have already been discussed.

Unique perhaps to the obese population may be their increased risk of radiation exposure. The basic premise in minimizing radiation exposure is time, distance, and shielding. Thus, injured patients or those with impaired mobility may be unable to move out of a contaminated area, thereby increasing their potential radiation exposure and dosage. If associated with trauma, obese patients with impaired wound healing are at increased risk of complications when irradiated because of the adverse interaction between trauma and radiation, that is, increasing radiation exposure worsens outcome in traumatized patients. Once diagnosed with acute radiation syndrome, these patients may require colony-stimulating factors and perhaps even stem cell transplantation.[35]

PALLIATIVE CARE AND MENTAL HEALTH SUPPORT

Increasingly, disaster settings require additional interventions beside typical medical and surgical support. Clearly, patients with underlying mental health disease, or those subject to the stresses imposed by a disaster, require important mental health support during the acute disaster phase as well as during recovery and reconstitution. The morbidly obese patients have been shown to be at increased risk for depression and hence, in addition to other increased resource needs during disasters, they also need mental health support.[36] Important also in disaster settings is the provision of pain management and palliative care, a requirement that is not unique to obese patients but nevertheless may pose challenges with additional health care staff attention and pharmacologic needs.[37]

DISASTER TRIAGE AND ALLOCATION OF SCARCE CRITICAL CARE RESOURCES

Although obese patients require increased support and resources, especially in a disaster setting, with appropriate planning and accommodation, most needs can be achieved through surging capacity of stuff, staff, and space. However, depending on the disaster and resource availability, tough triage decisions may be required when there are simply not enough resources to support all in need.

Given the additional resources, challenges, and scope of the problem in managing morbidly obese patients, under normal daily circumstances, there may be an inherent negative stereotype afforded to these patients. Many nurses believe the patients are not motivated to change their condition, and they do not believe they are effective in helping the patients achieve any behavioral change. Similarly, physicians have adverse opinions especially about the morbidly obese patients. The patients often view the health care community as biased against them, often disrespectful in the care they receive.[18]

Thus, faced with a disaster setting of limited resources and perhaps with some patient care bias in managing obese patients, a transparent process of triaging resources must be developed. Several models have recently been proposed in triaging hospital or ICU resources for nontrauma patients, so-called tertiary triage. Most models focus on use of the sequential organ failure assessment (SOFA) score. Through the use of an intensivist-led multidisciplinary triage team, patients in need of advanced clinical resources are evaluated for inclusion and then exclusion criteria and followed up using the SOFA score to determine illness severity and course. Patients with predicted high mortality or failure to improve, in this model, would be supported with palliative care and have their resources reallocated to other patients with greater chance of survival. Important to note is that none of the models specifically target patient weight as a criterion in determining need or exclusion; what counts is the severity of the illness.[38,39]

SUMMARY

Management of the morbidly obese patient under normal circumstances requires increased resources such as personnel, supplies, and special equipment. In the often resource-constrained setting of disasters, normal support to these patients may be jeopardized. In addition, their underlying condition with limited mobility and comorbidities may increase their likelihood of suffering harm depending on the type and tempo of the disaster. Morbidly obese patients are a special-needs population for whom necessary planning must be done to mitigate the effects of the disaster on them. Prior planning not only addresses appropriate care needs for these patients but also avoids crisis intervention during an event that might detract care and support from others during stressful times. In the end, such planning helps optimize the care for all.

REFERENCES

1. Hensrud D, Klein S. Extreme obesity: a new medical crisis in the United States. Mayo Clin Proc 2006;81(Suppl 10):S5–10.
2. Lurie N. H1N1 influenza, public health preparedness and health care reform. N Engl J Med 2009;361:843–5.
3. DeMaria E. Bariatric surgery for morbid obesity. N Engl J Med 2007;356: 2176–83.
4. McMahon M, Sarr M, Clark M, et al. Clinical management after bariatric surgery: value of a multidisciplinary approach. Mayo Clin Proc 2006;81(Suppl 10):S34–45.
5. Kahn CA, Oman JA, Rudkin SE, et al. Can ED staff accurately estimate the weight of adult patients? Am J Emerg Med 2007;25:307–12.
6. Block J, DeSalvo K, Fisher W. Are physicians equipped to address the obesity epidemic? Knowledge and attitudes of internal medicine residents. Prev Med 2003;36:669–75.
7. Berger E. Emergency departments shoulder challenges of providing care, providing dignity for the "super obese". Ann Emerg Med 2007;50(4):443–5.
8. Gougelet R. Modular medical systems (MEMS) for all types of catastrophic emergencies: a guide for community preparedness. Lebanon (NH): Dartmouth Medical School, New England Center for Emergency Preparedness; 2009.
9. Gifford A, Gougelet R. Intensive care unit microcosm within disaster medical response. In: Geiling J, editor. Fundamental disaster medicine. Mount Prospect (IL): Society of Critical Care Medicine; 2009. p. 2.1–2.14.
10. Gifford A, Spiro P. Augmenting critical care capacity during a disaster. In: Geiling J, editor. Fundamental disaster medicine. Mount Prospect (IL): Society of Critical Care Medicine; 2009. p. 3.1–3.10.
11. Jbeili C, Penet C, Jabre P, et al. [Out-of-hospital management characteristics of severe obese patients]. Ann Fr Anesth Réanim 2007;26:921–6 [in French].
12. Nguyen H, Schweitzer M, Magnuson T, et al. Bariatric surgery: the needs of the obese patient. Critical Connections Aug 2007;1:12. Available at: http://www.sccm.org/criticalconnections. Accessed July 14, 2010.
13. Grant P, Newcombe M. Emergency management of the morbidly obese. Emerg Med Australas 2004;16:309–17.
14. Rubinson R, Hick J, Curtis R, et al. Definitive care for the critically ill during a disaster: medical resources for surge capacity: from a Task Force for Mass Critical Care summit meeting, January 26–27, 2007, Chicago, IL. Chest 2008; 133:32S–50S.
15. Erstad B. Dosing of medications in morbidly obese patients in the intensive care unit setting. Intensive Care Med 2004;30:18–32.
16. Snow V, Barry P, Fitterman N, et al. Pharmacologic and surgical management of obesity in primary care: a clinical practice guideline from the American College of Physicians. Ann Intern Med 2005;142:525–31.

17. Devereaux A, Burns S, Gougelet R. Delivering acute care to chronically ill adults in shelters. In: Geiling J, editor. Fundamental disaster medicine. Mount Prospect (IL): Society of Critical Care Medicine; 2009. p. 11.1–11.14.
18. Devereaux A. Shelter medicine: beyond the first and second response. Chest Physician 2006;1:13.
19. Wolf L. The obese patient in the ED. Am J Nurs 2008;108:77–81.
20. Shaw L. Emergency preparedness & evacuation issues of the bariatric specialty population. Presented at National Bariatric Nurses Association Conference. Orlando (FL), November 6, 2009.
21. Tsismenakis A, Christophi C, Burress J. The obesity epidemic and future emergency responders. Obesity 2009;17:1648–50.
22. Haber C. Bariatric transport challenges: part 1. EMS Mag 2008;37:67–71.
23. Chinook information. Available at: http://en.wikipedia.org/wiki/CH-47_Chinook. Accessed July 14, 2010.
24. Pieracci F, Barie P, Pomp A. Critical care of the bariatric patient. Crit Care Med 2006;34:1796–804.
25. Meroz Y, Gozal Y. Management of the obese trauma patient. Anesthesiol Clin 2007;25:91–8.
26. Brown C, Neville A, Rhee P, et al. The impact of obesity on the outcomes of 1153 critically ill blunt trauma patients. J Trauma 2005;59:1048–51.
27. Winfield R, Delano M, Dixon D, et al. Differences in outcome between obese and nonobese patients following severe blunt trauma are not consistent with an early inflammatory genomic response. Crit Care Med 2010;38(1):51–8.
28. Hogue C, Stearns J, Colantuoni E, et al. The impact of obesity on outcomes after critical illness: a meta analysis. Intensive Care Med 2009;35:1152–70.
29. Sifri Z, Kim H, Lavery R, et al. The impact of obesity on the outcome of emergency intubation in trauma patients. J Trauma 2008;65:396–400.
30. Dries D, Bracco D, Razek T, et al. Conventional explosions and blast injuries. In: Geiling J, editor. Fundamental disaster medicine. Mount Prospect (IL): Society of Critical Care Medicine; 2009. p. 7.1–7.26.
31. Gottschlich M, Mayes T, Khoury J, et al. Significance of obesity on nutritional, immunologic, hormonal, and clinical outcome in burns. J Am Diet Assoc 1993; 93:1261–8.
32. Azocar R, Shaffer D. Disasters produced by natural phenomena. In: Geiling J, editor. Fundamental disaster medicine. Mount Prospect (IL): Society of Critical Care Medicine; 2009. p. 9.1–9.15.
33. Geiling J, Nicolais V, Susla G. Critical care management of chemical exposures. In: Geiling J, editor. Fundamental disaster medicine. Mount Prospect (IL): Society of Critical Care Medicine; 2009. p. 4.1–4.18.
34. Beigel J, Sandrock C. Intentional and natural outbreaks of infectious disease. In: Geiling J, editor. Fundamental disaster medicine. Mount Prospect (IL): Society of Critical Care Medicine; 2009. p. 5.1–5.30.
35. Amundson D, Bracco D, Parrish J. Critical care management of radiological emergencies. In: Geiling J, editor. Fundamental disaster medicine. Mount Prospect (IL): Society of Critical Care Medicine; 2009. p. 6.1–6.18.
36. Onyike C, Crum R, Hochang B, et al. Is obesity associated with major depression? Results from the third National Health and Nutrition Examination Survey. Am J Epidemiol 2003;158:1139–47.
37. Owens D. Palliative care and mental health issues. In: Geiling J, editor. Fundamental disaster medicine. Mount Prospect (IL): Society of Critical Care Medicine; 2009. p. 12.1–12.18.

38. Christian M, Farmer J, Young B. Disaster triage and allocation of scarce resources. In: Geiling J, editor. Fundamental disaster medicine. Mount Prospect (IL): Society of Critical Care Medicine; 2009. p. 13.1–13.18.
39. Devereaux A, Dichter J, Christian M, et al. Definitive care for the critically ill in a disaster: a framework for the allocation of scarce resources in mass critical care. Chest 2008;133:51S–66S.

Special Populations Critical Care Considerations of the Morbidly Obese Pregnant Patient

Marie R. Baldisseri, MD, FCCM[a],*,
Margaret D. Larkins-Pettigrew, MD, MEd, MPPM[b],*

KEYWORDS

- Morbidly obese • Obese • Pregnancy • Critical care
- Parturient

The incidence of obesity is increasing in the United States and worldwide.[1,2] Nearly one-quarter of adults in the United States are obese, with a body mass index (BMI) of 30.[3,4] In the United States, an estimated 30% to 40% of all women are obese, according to the National Institutes of Health consensus definition of obesity as 20% over the patient's relative weight.[5,6] This statistic is even more alarming in specific populations, with approximately 50% of African American and Mexican American women reported to be obese in the United States.[7] Of women aged 25 to 44 years in the United States, 26% to 40% are obese.[8] A BMI greater than 28 for women is also considered obese, and greater than 35 to 40 is considered morbidly obese.

The number of obese and morbidly obese pregnant women is also increasing each year. Several definitions of obesity and morbid obesity exist for pregnant patients. In the gravid patient at term, morbid obesity has been defined as greater than 300 lb or at least 100 lb overweight.[9] Garbaciak and colleagues[10] defined morbid obesity in a pregnant woman as 150% above her ideal body weight. Super obese patients were

---

The authors received no funding for this work and have no financial conflict of interest to disclose. The opinions and assertions contained herein are those of the authors and do not necessarily reflect the views or position the academic institutions with which the authors are affiliated.

[a] Department of Critical Care Medicine, University of Pittsburgh Medical Center, 613 Scaife Hall, 3550 Terrace Street, Pittsburgh, PA 15238, USA
[b] Department of Obstetrics, Gynecology and Reproductive Sciences, MacDonald Women's, Case Western University Medical Center, 11100 Euclid Avenue, Suite 7128, Cleveland, OH 44106, USA
* Corresponding authors.
E-mail addresses: baldisserimr@ccm.upmc.edu; Margaret.larkins-Pettigrew@uhhospitals.org

defined by Mason and colleagues[11] as those exceeding 225% of ideal body weight (ie, >123 kg and a BMI >46). Despite the many definitions of morbid obesity in the parturient, the prevalence of obesity in women of childbearing years is dramatically increasing among most ethnic and cultural populations. Recent estimates show that in the United States, 18.5% to 38.3% of pregnant women are obese, a 30% increase in the past 10 years.[12]

Mortality and disease risk increase exponentially with the degree of obesity.[13,14] Although obesity, and in particular morbid obesity, are associated with infertility, many obese women become pregnant. Obesity and morbid obesity result in significant risks to both the mother and the fetus. Obesity during pregnancy increases maternal hypertension, diabetes mellitus, preeclampsia, and anesthesia complications during labor and delivery.[9,15,16] Pregnant patients are at increased risk for obstetric complications and medical problems from the pathophysiologic changes associated with normal pregnancy. These risks to both the mother and fetus are significantly magnified when the parturient is obese or morbidly obese.

Pregnancy-related diseases and medical complications in the morbidly obese patient include systemic hypertension, diabetes, increased pulmonary and systemic venous thromboembolism, postpartum hemorrhage, wound infections, and urinary and genital tract infections. Obesity worsens perinatal outcomes as a direct result of maternal conditions, which include hypertension, diabetes mellitus, coronary disease, respiratory problems, and thromboembolic disease.[10,16,17] These prepregnant maternal disease states are often exacerbated during the pregnancy and the labor and delivery by the normal physiologic stresses associated with pregnancy. Some of these maternal medical conditions can present de novo during pregnancy and may be unmasked by the additional physiologic alterations of pregnancy.

Morbid obesity is an independent risk factor for adverse perinatal outcomes.[17–19] Obese pregnant patients have an increased number of antepartum stillbirths, especially at term, and spontaneous abortions and miscarriages. Stillbirths increase twofold in the presence of maternal obesity. Fetal complications and congenital anomalies as a result of maternal obesity include macrosomia and birth defects, particularly neural tube defects such as spina bifida.[20] These women have a much higher incidence of neonates with lower Apgar scores, higher birth weights, intrauterine growth retardation.[21] Several studies have shown an increase in cardiac defects in pregnancies complicated by obesity.[22,23] An increase is also seen in orofacial clefts, club foot, and abdominal wall defects. Craniofacial and musculoskeletal defects are increased threefold when pregnancy is complicated by both obesity and diabetes mellitus.

Other delivery complications include meconium, late decelerations, and shoulder dystocia.[10] Obese pregnant patients have a higher prevalence of gestational diabetes associated with an increased Cesarean section delivery rate and large birthweight babies.[17] Caesarean delivery risk is increased by 50% in overweight women and is more than double for obese women compared with women with normal BMI.[12] Both maternal and fetal death rates are increased, particularly in parturients who are morbidly obese at baseline. Obesity increases the risk of death during pregnancy because of risk factors such as advanced age, diabetes, hypertension, thromboembolic disease, and infection.[24–27] Morbidity increases in obese pregnant women postoperatively after Cesarean section, with higher rates of wound infections, dehiscence, and thromboembolic events.[28,29] Morbidity and mortality also increases during labor and delivery and the administration of anesthesia in the pregnant obese patient.[25–27,30,31]

PATHOPHYSIOLOGY OF PREGNANCY AND OBESITY

Many of the normal physiologic changes associated with pregnancy and labor and delivery may be additive, with many of the abnormal physiologic changes observed also in the morbidly obese nonpregnant patient. These deleterious alterations are aggravated when the morbidly obese patient becomes pregnant and is now faced with the additional physiologic stresses of pregnancy. The obese pregnant woman is also more susceptible to pregnancy-related complications, such as preeclampsia, hypertension, and diabetes. Hood and Dewan[9] observed a 14-fold increase in the incidence of hypertension among obese parturients who weighed more than 300 lb at delivery.

Obesity results in a two- to eightfold increase in the incidence of insulin-dependent diabetes during pregnancy.[10,32,33] The association of disease states frequently associated with morbid obesity, such as diabetes, hypertension, and respiratory problems, further complicate pregnancy in the morbidly obese patient, increasing both maternal and fetal morbidity and mortality.

Cardiovascular Changes

Changes in blood volume and cardiovascular function are significant adaptive mechanisms that accommodate the increased metabolic needs of both the mother and the fetus during pregnancy, and labor and delivery. Blood volume increases exponentially and reaches 30% to 50% above prepartum values by term. Cardiac output increases up to 50% above prepregnancy values by the 24th week of gestation, and then plateaus until labor and delivery. Cardiac output increases primarily as a result of increased stroke volume during the first two trimesters, and from an increase in the heart rate during the third trimester until term.

Oxygen consumption increases up to 20% to 30% at term and up to 60% during labor and delivery as a result of the increased metabolic needs of both the mother and the fetus. Approximately 30 mL of blood are required per kilogram of adipose tissue.[34] The increased blood volume of the obese patient coupled with increased metabolic needs can increase myocardial demand and precipitate high-output cardiac failure in the morbidly obese. Cardiac failure in the obese can result in diastolic dysfunction, left atrial enlargement, and left ventricular hypertrophy.[35]

Remodeling of the heart with four-chamber enlargement is also seen in normal pregnancy. Hemodynamic studies in normal pregnancy have shown increases in cardiac output, left ventricular stroke work, and oxygen consumption.[36,37] Filling pressures are unchanged during pregnancy, despite a larger blood volume, because of decreased systemic and pulmonary resistances accommodating higher volumes at normal vascular pressures.[36,37] Healthy pregnant women can tolerate the cardiovascular and hemodynamic effects associated with pregnancy. Patients with mild to moderate cardiovascular disease have a higher incidence of heart failure and arrhythmias during pregnancy, but overall mortality is unchanged. Patients with either primary or secondary pulmonary hypertension or right-to-left shunts have maternal mortality rates as high as 50% and poor fetal outcomes.

Many of these changes described in pregnant patients are also seen in the nonpregnant morbidly obese patient, such as decreased total peripheral resistance, increased cardiac diameter, increased cardiac output secondary to larger stroke volumes, increased right and left ventricular stroke work, and increased oxygen consumption.[38] These changes are further amplified in the morbidly obese patient during pregnancy. A study of obese hypertensive patients by Mabie and colleagues[39] showed these patients to have increased left ventricular mass and diastolic dysfunction but relatively normal systolic function. The authors suggested that this reflected volume overload with inadequate left ventricular relaxation.

Respiratory Changes

The major pulmonary changes that occur in pregnancy include an increase in tidal volume of approximately 40%, a decrease in functional residual capacity (FRC) of 25%, and a substantial increase of up to 30% in oxygen consumption. Total lung capacity decreases only minimally in pregnancy.[40] The decreased FRC and increased oxygen consumption diminish the oxygen reserve of the mother and increase the hypoxic risk to both the mother and the fetus in the event of maternal hypoventilation or apnea. The 30% to 40% increase in minute ventilation, primarily as a result of an increased tidal volume, offsets the oxygen requirements that increase by approximately 30 to 40 mL/min in pregnancy. Increased minute ventilation in the nonobese pregnant woman normally increases ao_2 from 104 to 108 mm Hg, in contrast with a more modest increase in the pregnant obese woman, in whom the Pao_2 increases 80 to 85 mm Hg over her nonpregnant state.[41] The increase in minute ventilation results in a mild compensated respiratory alkalosis, with a decline in the $Paco_2$ to 28 to 32 mm Hg. The pH does not change because of renal compensation, which results in a decrease in serum bicarbonate concentration.

Preexisting pulmonary changes of the morbidly obese pregnant patient compound the pulmonary alterations of the parturient. Decreased total respiratory compliance of both the chest wall and the lung is seen in the morbidly obese patient. This occurrence coupled with the mass loading of the lungs results in a decrease in the FRC from a decreased expiratory reserve volume (ERV). This decrease in ERV is further aggravated by changes in position, especially in the supine position. The supine position further decreases the FRC because of cephalad displacement of the diaphragm by the abdominal contents. The FRC and the tidal volume may fall below the closing capacity, leading to alveolar collapse and further exacerbate ventilation–perfusion mismatching. The reduction in FRC and the increased metabolic demands of the morbidly obese further increase the hypoxic risk to the mother and the fetus. Pelosi and colleagues[42] found that an increased BMI leads to a proportionate decrease in FRC and lung compliance resulting in increased work of breathing.

Eng and colleagues[41] measured lung volumes in obese pregnant women during the third trimester and postpartum. He found lung volumes to be comparable to nonobese pregnant women, but FRC was decreased in the pregnant obese women, although less than expected compared with normal controls. The FRC of normal patients decreases by approximately 20% after induction of anesthesia. In morbidly obese patients, the FRC may decrease as much as 50%, causing microatelectasis with ventilation/perfusion mismatching and an increase in the alveolar–arterial gradient. Intrapulmonary shunt will increase from 2% to 5% in nonobese patients to 10% to 20% in obese patients.

Morbidly obese patients frequently have thoracolumbar lordosis and modified thoracic curve that may be further worsened during pregnancy. The large gravid uterus and abdomen decrease rib movement and further restrict lung expansion. Excess chest wall and abdominal fat further limit respiratory excursion. Pulmonary complications that can occur during pregnancy, such as pneumonia, pulmonary edema, and pulmonary embolism, will increase the work of breathing in the obese pregnant patient, who may already have underlying significant pulmonary alterations as a result of obesity.

In severe restrictive lung disease as seen in the adult respiratory distress syndrome, the limitation of lung expansion associated with both pregnancy and morbid obesity may prompt expeditious delivery of the fetus while on mechanical ventilation to more efficiently and effectively expand the lungs. Depending on gestational age and fetal lung maturity, this may place the fetus at risk for complications associated with low birthweight and early gestational age.

Significant intrinsic lung disease associated with hypoxemia and hypercarbia from alveolar hypoventilation in morbidly obese pregnant patients places both the mother and fetus at significant risk. These changes are seen with increased prevalence in the obese patient who has obstructive sleep apnea and obstructive lung disease. Maternal arterial Pco_2 is in the range of 28 to 32 mm Hg because of the mild respiratory alkalosis. A pregnant patient with a Pco_2 of 38 mm Hg and Pao_2 of 70 mm Hg has evidence of acute respiratory distress. Transfer of CO_2 across the placenta is dependent on a Pco_2 difference of 10 mm Hg between fetal and maternal umbilical veins. If maternal hypercapnia occurs, this will quickly result in fetal respiratory acidosis. Acidosis shifts the fetal oxygen dissociation curve to the right, decreasing the ability of oxygen to bind to fetal hemoglobin.

Airway obstruction with obstructive sleep apnea resulting in significant hypercarbia and hypoxemia can cause complications in the morbidly obese parturient. Sleep-disordered breathing, with increases in apnea, oxygen desaturation, and snoring times, is more common in obese pregnant women. This condition may predispose to intrauterine fetal growth restriction in the offspring, and hypertensive disorders and increased cardiovascular risk in the mothers. Normal airway changes as a result of increased estrogen levels in the parturient show increased mucosal edema, with capillary engorgement and hyperemia that may be problematic because this may lead to difficulty in visualizing the landmarks of the upper airway. Airway edema can be further increased by a prolonged second stage of labor and in preeclamptic patients.

Although airway edema and hyperemia are observed in the pregnant patient, they do not impact airflow rates. Pregnancy itself is associated with lower oncotic pressures. The decreased oncotic pressure is more pronounced in the preeclamptic patient, leading to upper airway edema.[43] For this reason, a smaller-diameter endotracheal tube is usually necessary when intubating a pregnant patient with advanced gestation. A progression in Mallampati classification in advanced pregnancy has been reported.[44] These anatomic changes may further exacerbate and complicate the situation in obese pregnant patients who require endotracheal intubation.

Hematologic Changes

In pregnancy, a disproportionate increase in plasma volume of 40% to 60% occurs with only a 25% increase in red cell mass at term, resulting in a dilutional anemia with a hemoglobin concentration of approximately 11 g/dL at 24 weeks. This event may be offset by the polycythemia seen in morbidly obese patients as compensation for a baseline hypoxemia. Plasma concentrations of all clotting factors except XI, XIII, and antithrombin III increase during pregnancy, although no change occurs in coagulation testing and bleeding times. However, these changes result in a hypercoagulable state that, in association with increased procoagulant proteins, venous stasis, and vessel wall trauma, significantly increase the risk for thromboembolic disease.

Obesity is associated with increased levels of factor VII and VIII, von Willebrand factor, and fibrinogen, which also increase the risk of thromboembolism. Both pregnancy and obesity additively increase the risk of venous and pulmonary thromboembolism, placing the obese parturient at even greater risk for either or both of these complications. Estimates of the age-adjusted incidence of venous thromboembolism range from 4 to 50 times higher in pregnant than in nonpregnant women, with an absolute incidence rate of 1 in 500 to 2000 pregnancies (0.025%–0.10%).[45,46] A direct correlation exists between the incidence of venous thromboembolism and increasing body weight.[29] A sixfold increase in the incidence of pulmonary emboli has been seen in patients with a BMI of 35 compared with those with a BMI of 22.[29]

Endocrine Changes

Pregnancy alters maternal endocrine metabolism and hormonal feedback mechanisms, although the incidence of severe endocrine abnormalities during pregnancy is relatively uncommon. However, disease manifestations may be difficult to distinguish from the normal hypermetabolic state of pregnancy. Thyroid disorders are commonly encountered during pregnancy. Three major factors alter maternal thyroid physiology in pregnancy: significant alterations in iodide physiology, the stimulation of the thyroid by human chorionic gonadotropin, and an increase in thyroxine-binding globulin. Hyperthyroidism occurs in 0.2% of pregnancies.[47] Thyroid storm is a medical emergency associated with 25% mortality for both the mother and the fetus. It generally occurs in previously undiagnosed hyperthyroid patients and can be precipitated by intrapartum or postpartum infections or by labor and delivery of the parturient.

Hypothyroidism occurs in 2.5% of pregnancies.[48] The incidence is higher in women with type 1 diabetes who have microvascular complications. Diabetes mellitus occurs more frequently in obese patients. Decreased insulin sensitivity can be seen in obese patients, particularly in those with upper-body obesity.[49] Insulin sensitivity seems to decline after 12 to 14 weeks of gestation, with progression to severe insulin resistance during the third trimester.[50]

Gastrointestinal Changes

Because of the large gravid uterus with advanced gestational age and a concomitant delay in gastric emptying and decrease in lower esophageal sphincter tone from increased progesterone levels, the parturient is at higher risk for pulmonary aspiration of gastric contents. Pregnant patients have increased intra-abdominal pressure because of the expanding gravid uterus, which increases their risk of aspiration. Obese patients are reported to have delayed gastric emptying and low gastric pH[51,52] are also at increased risk of aspiration, which is further increased if they become pregnant.

Intensive Care Unit Care of the Obese Pregnant Patient

Increased morbidity and mortality and length of intensive care unit (ICU) stay of obese patients may result from the increased physiologic strain and stress on the cardiopulmonary system from both the obese state and from obesity-related comorbidities. These increases are also seen with obese pregnant patients. Considering the myriad of physiologic changes associated with morbid obesity and pregnancy, the expected complications, morbidity, and mortality increase significantly.

The overall prevalence of obstetric patients who require ICU admission and critical care management during their pregnancy is less than 1% of all ICU admissions.[3,53,54] ICU admissions occur in approximately 0.5% of all pregnant women.[3,53,54] The mortality rate of critically ill obstetric patients ranges from 12% to 20%.[55] Critically ill pregnant patients present unique challenges to the practitioner who must have a complete understanding and a good working knowledge of the normal physiologic changes associated with pregnancy, the period of labor and delivery, and the postpartum period. In addition to understanding the normal and abnormal physiology of pregnancy, the practitioner must have a clear understanding of the specific changes associated with the morbidly obese patient.

The physiologic changes associated with both pregnancy and morbid obesity, especially during critical illness, result in complex maternal pathophysiology that presents a difficult and unique challenge to the practitioner. Therefore, these patients must be managed with a multidisciplinary team of clinicians. The expertise of intensivists, anesthesiologists, and maternal-fetal medicine obstetricians will be required to treat these complex patients to achieve good maternal and fetal outcomes.

The most common causes of ICU admission are postpartum hemorrhage, respiratory disorders, and complications of severe preeclampsia. The highest mortality in developed countries is secondary to pulmonary embolism, amniotic fluid embolism, and trauma. In developing countries, postpartum hemorrhage remains the principal cause of maternal death. The more common causes of critical illness in pregnant patients are usually precipitated by the physiologic stresses of pregnancy, such as underlying maternal cardiac or respiratory diseases. A slightly lesser number of patients with critical illness are those with conditions that are unique to pregnancy, such as severe preeclampsia, amniotic fluid embolism, and postpartum hemorrhage.

Because critical illness in the morbidly obese has been extensively described elsewhere in this issue, this section will focus mainly on maternal oxygenation, ventilation, hemodynamics, and maternal resuscitation associated with critical illness of the pregnant patient. Respiratory illnesses are a frequent reason why pregnant patients are admitted to the ICU. The causes of respiratory failure in the obstetric patient are similar to those in the nonpregnant patient. These conditions include respiratory failure as a result of pneumonia; acute respiratory distress syndrome (ARDS) from sepsis or trauma; pulmonary embolism; preeclampsia and pulmonary edema; peripartum cardiomyopathy and left heart failure; tocolytic-induced pulmonary edema; and acute asthmatic exacerbations.

Asthma is the most common respiratory condition complicating pregnancy, and is associated with increased maternal and fetal morbidity and mortality.[55] Systemic corticosteroids for the treatment of severe asthma in the parturient have been recommended by the American Academy of Obstetricians and Gynecologists and the American College of Allergy, Asthma and Immunology.[56] Two small studies have shown a positive outcome in pregnant patients who were treated with inhaled corticosteroids.[57,58]

Pulmonary edema is caused by a multiplicity of conditions associated with pregnancy. The diagnosis and treatment of pregnant patients with pulmonary edema are not much different from those of nonpregnant patients, particularly if the pulmonary edema is cardiogenic in nature. Pulmonary edema associated with severe preeclampsia may result from several mechanisms, including lower oncotic pressure (even in the absence of increased hydrostatic pressures) and increased cardiac permeability. In these complex patients, especially if the preeclampsia is complicated by severe oliguria, invasive hemodynamic monitoring may be required if the pulmonary edema does not respond to diuresis and judicious fluid management.[59]

Invasive monitoring for diagnosis and management may also be required for specific obstetric-related conditions such as New York Heart Association (NYHA) III or IV cardiac disease, amniotic fluid embolism, and primary or secondary pulmonary hypertension, especially as a result of significant mitral stenosis.

The management of bacterial and viral pneumonias seen in pregnancy is similar to that for nonpregnant patients, although mechanical ventilation management may be more complicated in those who develop ARDS as a sequela because of the severe restrictive lung disease. In addition, obese patients have been found to be ventilator-dependent for longer periods than nonobese patients.[3] Experts have postulated that the pregnant patient may be more susceptible to infections, although no firm data support this.

Regardless of the specific pulmonary cause, the greatest danger to the parturient is the increased hypoxic risk to the mother and the fetus as a result of maternal hypoventilation or apnea. The 25° head-up position has been recommended to optimize preoxygenation in pregnant women and morbidly obese patients.[60] This positioning may help improve gas exchange and reduce ventilation–perfusion mismatching in pregnant patients and obese patients. Even with adequate preoxygenation, oxygen saturations decrease significantly faster in pregnant patients and morbidly obese patients,[61,62] which mandates careful monitoring and titration of oxygenation in the pregnant patient.

Because maternal oxygenation is shared by the mother and fetal uteroplacental unit, it has been recommended that higher FiO_2 levels be administered to the mother to prevent precipitous decreases in oxygen saturation and the possibility of precipitating fetal anoxia.

The indications for intubation and ventilation are the same for pregnant patients and nonpregnant patients. The use of noninvasive ventilation (NIV) has not been well described in pregnancy, and caution must be exercised with its use because of the increased airway edema and increased risk of aspiration. NIV in the pregnant patient should be reserved for those who are awake and alert and protecting their airway. However, as a temporizing measure, it may be successful in preventing endotracheal intubation in some instances.

Endotracheal intubation in pregnant women is usually more difficult because of the airway edema and hyperemia. The failure rate for intubations in pregnant patients is 1 in 280 compared with 1 in 2330 in the general surgical population.[63] Failure to intubate may be associated with higher risk for poor fetal and maternal outcomes. Anesthesia-related mortality is a significant cause of maternal mortality in the United States.[64]

Ventilation of the pregnant patient is similar to that of nonpregnant patients, except that it should be directed to a slightly lower Pco_2 level because the normal pregnant state is mild respiratory alkalosis with Pco_2 levels of 28 to 32 mm Hg. Excessive hyperventilation will lead to uterine vasoconstriction with decreased placental and fetal perfusion and subsequent fetal distress. Pco_2 levels of 55 to 60 mm Hg seem to be well tolerated by the fetus, but more severe hypercapnia and hypoventilation could precipitate fetal acidemia and distress. Treatment with bicarbonate may improve maternal and fetal acidemia in this instance.

The patient with ARDS presents unique challenges to the practitioner, because the restrictive lung disease of ARDS is further complicated by anatomic restriction of the pregnant state with decreased chest wall and abdominal wall compliance. The ideal body weight of a pregnant patient is unclear, but based on the ARDSnet protocol, this rule should be followed to calculate and deliver an adequate tidal volume but prevent barotrauma and volutrauma in these patients.[65]

The goal of low tidal volume ventilation is to avoid overdistension of the lung. Because total lung capacity is relatively unchanged between the pregnant and nonpregnant state, the recommendation to use lower tidal volumes of 6 mL/kg seems reasonable. Calculation of the ideal tidal volume is based on the ideal body weight more complex when the pregnant patient is morbidly obese. Delivery of the fetus may be required in those instances, particularly in patients with ARDS in whom the gravid uterus is further restricting lung expansion. However, the therapeutic effect of this has been questioned.[66]

Sedatives and muscle paralytics may be required during pregnancy, especially for patients who require endotracheal intubation and continued mechanical ventilation. Narcotic analgesics are not associated with specific fetal anomalies. Propofol has been used as an induction agent for Cesarean deliveries, but no data exist on its prolonged use in pregnancy. Caution should be exercised when using benzodiazepines because these drugs freely cross the placenta and may accumulate in the fetus. Midazolam and lorazepam cross the placenta to a lesser degree than diazepam and are not associated with the risk of cleft lip and palate seen with the use of diazepam early in pregnancy. Neuromuscular blocking agents also cross the placenta but do not seem to have lasting clinical effects on the fetus.

Hypotension management in the parturient requires particular attention to body position and volume status. Untreated maternal hypotension is obviously detrimental to the mother and fetus. Proper positioning of the mother in the left lateral decubitus position, or at least with the right hip elevated, is required to optimize maternal cardiac output and preload. Vasoactive agents may be required if fluid resuscitation is unsuccessful, as in nonpregnant patients. Fluid resuscitation must be administered adequately because the addition of vasoconstricting agents will compromise utero-placental flow if vasoconstriction is imposed on an insufficient circulating volume. All vasoactive agents have the potential to constrict uterine vessels and reduce blood flow to the placenta and fetus despite improving maternal blood pressures. Placental blood flow and uterine perfusion pressure are directly proportional to maternal systemic blood pressure and cardiac output.

Little literature exists on the choice of vasoactive agents for pregnant patients with persistent shock. Most available studies address transient use of vasopressors for hypotension associated with spinal anesthesia or in the operative setting. Pregnant patients seem to be more susceptible to hypotension after a sympathetic block with spinal or epidural anesthesia.[67] Other causes of hypotension in the pregnant patient are the same as those in the general population and include sepsis, hypovolemia, anaphylaxis, and cardiogenic shock.

Animal studies suggest that ephedrine, a sympathomimetic agent, is least likely to cause uterine vasoconstriction, and remains the recommended first-line agent for pregnant patients, particularly after spinal or epidural anesthesia-related hypotension. Phenylephrine and metaraminol are also favored for short-term use of maternal hypotension. Recent reports show that ephedrine may be associated with higher heart rates and increased rates of fetal acidosis compared with phenylephrine.[68,69] Morbidly obese patient may not respond to adrenergic receptor activation, because the obese myocardium has a decreased relative number of adrenergic receptors and the response to ß-blockers and adrenergics may be attenuated.[70] These changes may play a significant role in the critically ill obese pregnant woman seriously ill with heart failure or hemodynamic instability seen commonly in sepsis, when the use of ß-blockers or adrenergic agents may be required. Norepinephrine has also been suggested for persistent shock in pregnant patients in the ICU setting, but no specific data support or refute this.

Diagnostic studies are usually mandated for care of the critically ill pregnant patient. Radiographic examinations should never be delayed or deferred because the patient is pregnant. Estimated fetal radiation exposure for most diagnostic radiographic studies is low and acceptable, especially when an abdominal lead shield and a well-collimated x-ray beam are used. Abdominal and pelvic CT scans are associated with the highest fetal radiation exposures, of up to 5 rads. Teratogenicity does not occur until the total fetal radiation exposure over the course of gestation exceeds 10 rads. Cumulative exposure to less than 5 rads throughout the pregnancy has been shown to increase the risk of childhood leukemias.[71] The risk benefit–ratio should always be considered when ordering a radiographic test in pregnant patients, although the risks are minimal with judicious planning.

Care should be taken during any radiographic examination of the parturient that requires that the patient be supine. It is important that the time lying supine is minimized or that the patient remain in the left lateral decubitus position during the examination. This positioning is to prevent hemodynamic compromise from compression of the aorta and the inferior vena cava by the large gravid uterus. Cardiac output in the pregnant patient can decrease by 25% in the supine position.

Severity of Illness Scoring Systems in Pregnancy

The APACHE II (Acute Physiology and Chronic Health Evaluation), SAPS II (Simplified Acute Physiology Score), and MPM II scores (Mortality Probability Model) have all been used to predict mortality of critically ill patients. However, these scoring systems are not specific for the pregnant patient and may be inaccurate for predicting in this population. Normal pregnancy physiologic variables, such as increased heart rate and decreased hematocrit, lead to higher APACHE scores, whereas specific abnormal variables, such as hemolysis, thrombocytopenia, and elevated liver function tests, are not rated as abnormal but signify significant maternal compromise in severe preeclampsia. APACHE II has overestimated maternal mortality in several studies.[72–75] Two studies have found that APACHE II and SAPS accurately predicted mortality in obstetric patients with medical disorders but were less reliable in patients with primary obstetric disorders.[74,76] Bhagwanjee and colleagues[77] found the Glasgow Coma Scale to be a good predictor of outcome compared with APACHE in preeclamptic patients. Given the variable reliability of these scoring systems in pregnancy, some interest has been shown in using ICU admission as the single variable that identifies patients with severe morbidity that may lead to increased mortality.[78]

Studies have observed similar rates of mortality in pregnant and nonpregnant critically ill patients using APACHE II, SAPS II, and MPM II scores[3,77] Pregnancy itself does not seem to increase mortality beyond the expected mortality rate of the critical illness. However, the morbidly obese patient will have increased mortality based on her degree of obesity rather than from the pregnancy.

Active Management of Labor of the Critically Ill Morbidly Obese Patient

The ICU is often where critically ill patients give birth. The gravid uterus and the fetal requirements can contribute to the instability of an already compromised mother. Careful and prudent decision making is the key to ensure a healthy fetus while limiting the normal stress associated with this event. The approach to the management of morbidly obese patients during parturition is always a challenge, but a vaginal delivery is ideal. The five major concerns during the intrapartum period are adequate pain management, induction of labor, augmentation of labor, shortening of the second stage of labor, and management of complications associated with the third stage of labor, such as hemorrhage, infection, deep vein thrombosis, and hypertensive disease. Special consideration and management of maternal comorbidities, such as diabetes, cardiovascular, and hypertensive disease, greatly influence the neonatal outcome of patients who may encounter issues such as intrauterine growth restriction, macrosomia, and risk for shoulder dystocia, fetal hyperbilirubinemia, and hypoglycemia.

Physiology of Labor

Labor consists of synchronized myometrial activity that results in effacement and dilatation of the uterine cervix. Several hormones are involved in the parturitional cascade, including prostaglandins, progesterone, estrogen, oxytocin, corticotrophin-releasing hormone, parathyroid hormone–related peptide, luteinizing hormone, relaxin, and cytokines.[79–81] These hormones may experience some alteration in expression resulting in early onset of labor, dysfunctional labor, or post-date deliveries.[82–86]

Intravenous Sedation

Labor is a physically, mentally, and emotionally stressful event. Pain relief and relaxation of pelvic muscles can assist in the progression of labor. The use of sedatives such as nubain and stadol can assist in initial pain management. These agents must be used with caution because of maternal and fetal respiratory side effects. In the morbidly obese patient, the dosage of these agents may need to be modified for effect secondary to decreased volume.[87] These agents should not be given if delivery is anticipated within 2 hours of administration. Maternal to placental transmission may result in fetal respiratory depression and delay in fetal transition.

Anesthetic Management

Pain during labor is an added stressor that must be managed but is often a challenge for the morbidly obese patient. Lumbar epidural analgesia with dilute bupivacaine and fentanyl is the optimal choice. This technique minimizes motor blockade but an increased failure rate is documented second to greater depth of the epidural space.[88,89] Placing the epidural while the patient is in the sitting position allows landmark anatomic structures to be located if the patient can tolerate this position, but it increases the distance between the skin and the space. This distance is minimized with flexion but longer needles and at times ultrasound guidance must be used. Once placed, the catheter may be dislodged on movement to the lateral decubitus position because of redistribution of the soft tissue of the back.[89] Therefore, it is recommended that the catheter be placed with the patient in the sitting position, and secured before movement. Morbidly obese patients are also at risk for a high spinal because of a decrease in cerebrospinal fluid volume.[90,91] Timing for placement of the epidural is critical either with or without medication dosing. The epidural will offer ideal pain relief and could potentially avoid the need for general anesthesia.

Induction and Augmentation of Labor

If the critically ill patient would benefit from delivery of a mature fetus and spontaneous onset of labor has not occurred, induction of labor may be required. Numerous combination methods may be used to manage this first stage of labor. Mechanical methods used for induction such as membrane stripping, cervical Foley bulb placement, osmotic dilators (Laminaria japonicum), and amniotomy have minimal contraindications for the mother.[92,93]

Cervical ripening agents and Pitocin are the gold standards if labor is not spontaneous and progressive. Prostaglandin E2 agents, such as prepidil (dinoprostone) intracervical gel of 0.5 mg for two doses or cervidil (dinoprostone) intravaginal 10-mg dosing, have limited side effects such as uterine hyperstimulation and induced fetal hypoxia.[94,95] Maternal complications are minimal. Misoprostol (Cytotec), a prostaglandin E1 analog in 25 to 50 μg tablets, which is also administered vaginally, orally, or sublingually, should be avoided because of an increased risk of uterine hyperstimulation. The inability to remove this product to help reverse this complications and ultimate fetal hypoxia makes this agent least desirable.[95]

Pitocin, an octopeptide and short-acting uterotonic, works to induce and augment the first and second stages of labor. Pitocin concentration of 10 to 40 units in 1000 mL of isotonic solution is equal to 10 to 40 mU/mL. Most providers believe the maximum amount of Pitocin is that which is most effective, but a maximum of 30 units over a 12-hour period is recommended. The short half-life of 5 minutes and the ability to rapidly reverse its effects makes this agent ideal as a method to actively manage labor. Pitocin, however, has side effects that may influence hemodynamic stability secondary to its known maternal cardiovascular and pulmonary effects, and causes untoward fetal effects. Close monitoring by seasoned labor and delivery staff is essential.[92–94]

Active Management of the Second Stage of Labor

Managing the second stage of labor can be an active or passive process for the provider. Many times the neonate must be delivered using vacuum extraction or forceps to shorten the second stage of labor.[96] The American Congress of Obstetricians and Gynecologists recommends shortening the second stage of labor as indicated for maternal benefit and when immediate or potential fetal compromise is suspected. Cardiovascular or respiratory challenges that may be further exacerbated by the act of pushing may warrant vaginal instrumentation. In the morbidly obese patient, the risks to the fetus during a vaginal delivery, such as shoulder dystocia and intracranial hemorrhage, may mandate a caesarean delivery.

The Third Stage of Labor

The major complication associated with the third stage of labor is postpartum hemorrhage. The cause of a postpartum hemorrhage can be uterine atony or cervical and vaginal lacerations. Contributing factors may be prolonged use of Pitocin, magnesium sulfate use, chorioamnionitis, or multiple gestations. The management of postpartum hemorrhage in morbidly obese patients is challenging because of the inability to obtain adequate external and internal uterine massage and manually remove retained products. The ability to visualize tears for repair may be compromised by significant redundant vaginal tissues. Other complications include infection and deep venous thrombosis.[97]

SUMMARY

The critically ill pregnant patient poses a unique challenge to the clinician, requiring a thorough understanding of normal and abnormal maternal and fetal physiology associated with pregnancy. The morbidly obese patient presents even greater challenges to the clinician, and morbidity and mortality are proportionately increased. Because increased numbers of obese pregnant women are now admitted to ICUs, practitioners must be aware of the physiology associated with both pregnancy and obesity. A multidisciplinary approach is imperative to prevent both maternal and fetal morbidity and mortality for these very complex patients, especially when they are admitted to the ICU with critical illness.

REFERENCES

1. Mokad AH, Serdula MK, Dietz WH, et al. The spread of the obesity epidemic in the United States, 1991–1998. JAMA 1999;282:1319–22.
2. Centers for Disease Control and Prevention. U.S. Obesity Trends: Trends by State 1985–2009. Available at: http://www.cdc.gov/obesity/trends.html. Accessed June 1, 2010.
3. El-Sohl A, Sikka P, Bozkanat E, et al. Morbid obesity in the medical ICU. Chest 2001;120:1989–97.

4. World Health Organization. Obesity: preventing and managing the global epidemic. Report of a WHO convention, Geneva, 1999. WHO technical report series 894, Geneva (Switzerland): World Health Organization; 2000.
5. National Institute of Health Consensus Development Conference Statement. Health implications of obesity. Ann Intern Med 1985;103:147–51.
6. Bray GA. Obesity. In: Fauci AS, Marlin JB, Braunwald E, et-al, editors. Harrison's principles of internal medicine. 14th edition. New York: McGraw-Hill; 1998. p. 454–62.
7. Flegal KM, Carroll MD, Ogden CL, et al. Prevalence and trends in obesity among US adults, 1999-2000. JAMA 2002;288:1723–7.
8. Centers for Disease Control and Prevention. Health United States, 2003. Available at: http://www.cdc.gov/nchs/data/hus/hus03.pdf. Accessed June 1, 2010.
9. Hood DD, Dewan DM. Anesthesia and obstetric outcome in morbidly obese parturients. Anesthesiology 1993;79:1210–8.
10. Garbaciak JJ, Richter M, Miller S, et al. Maternal weight and pregnancy complications. Am J Obstet Gynecol 1991;164:1306–10.
11. Mason E, Doherty C, Maher J, et al. Super obesity and gastric reduction procedure. Gastroenterol Clin North Am 1987;16:495–502.
12. Poobalan AS, Aucott LS, Gurung T, et al. Obesity as an independent risk factor for elective and emergency caesarean delivery in nulliparous women - systematic review and meta-analysis of cohort studies. Obes Rev 2009;10:28–35.
13. Strauss R. Operative risk of obesity. Surg Gynecol Obstet 1978;146:286–90.
14. Kral JC. Morbid obesity and related health risks. Ann Intern Med 1985;103:1043–7.
15. Johnson SR, Kolberg GH, Varner MW. Maternal obesity and pregnancy. Surg Gynecol Obstet 1987;164:431–7.
16. Baeten JM, Bukusi EA, Lambe M. Pregnancy complications and outcomes among overweight and obese nulliparous women. Am J Public Health 2001;91:436–40.
17. Sebire N, Jolly M, Harris J, et al. Maternal obesity and pregnancy outcome: a study of 287,213 pregnancies in London. Int J Obes Relat Metab Disord 2001;25:1175–82.
18. Kumari AS. Pregnancy outcome in women with morbid obesity. Int J Gynaecol Obstet 2001;73:101–7.
19. Cnattingius S, Bergstrom R, Lipworth L, et al. Prepregnancy weight and the risk of adverse pregnancy outcomes. N Engl J Med 1998;338:147–52.
20. Waller DK, Millis JL, Simpson JL, et al. Are obese women at higher risk for producing malformed offspring? Am J Obstet Gynecol 1994;170:541.
21. Perlow J, Morgan M, Montgomery D, et al. Perinatal outcome in pregnancy complicated by massive obesity. Am J Obstet Gynecol 1992;167:958–62.
22. Galtier-Dereure F, Boegner C, Bringer J. Obesity and pregnancy: complications and cost. Am J Clin Nutr 2000;71:1242S–8S.
23. Watkins ML, Botto LD. Maternal prepregnancy weight and congenital heart defects in the offspring. Epidemiology 2001;11:439–46.
24. Rochat R, Koonin L, Atrash A, et al. Maternal mortality in the United States: report from the maternal mortality collaborative. Obstet Gynecol 1988;72:91–7.
25. May W, Greiss F. Maternal mortality in North Carolina: a four year experience. Am J Obstet Gynecol 1989;161:555–61.
26. Endler G, Mariona F, Solol R, et al. Anesthesia-related mortality in Michigan 1972–1984. Am J Obstet Gynecol 1988;158:187–93.
27. Sachs B, Oriol N, Ostheimer G, et al. Anesthetic related maternal mortality 1954-1985. J Clin Anesth 1989;1:333–8.

28. Eichinger S, Hron G, Bialonczyk C, et al. Overweight, obesity, and the risk of recurrent venous thromboembolism. Arch Intern Med 2008;168:1678–83.

29. Kabrhel C, Varraso R, Goldhaber SZ, et al. Prospective study of BMI and the risk of pulmonary embolism in women. Obesity (Silver Spring) 2009;17:2040–6.

30. Adams JP, Murphy PG. Obesity in anaesthesia and intensive care. Br J Anaesth 2000;85:91–108.

31. Hawkins JL, Koonin LM, Palmer SK, et al. Anesthesia-related deaths during obstetric delivery in the United States, 1979–1990. Anesthesiology 1997;86:277–84.

32. Kliegman R, Gross T. Perinatal problems of the obese mother and her infant. Obstet Gynecol 1985;66:299–306.

33. Gross T, Sokol R, King K. Obesity and pregnancy: risk and outcome. Obstet Gynecol 1980;56:446–50.

34. Alexander JK. The cardiomyopathy of obesity. Prog Cardiovasc Dis 1985;27: 325–33.

35. Movahed MR, Saito Y. Obesity is associated with left atrial enlargement, E/A reversal and left ventricular hypertrophy. Exp Clin Cardiol 2008;13:89–91.

36. Clark SL, Cotton DB, Lee W, et al. Central hemodynamic assessment of normal term pregnancy. Am J Obstet Gynecol 1989;161:1439–42.

37. Campos O, Andrade JL, Bocanegra J, et al. Physiologic multivalvular regurgitation during pregnancy: a longitudinal Doppler echocardiographic study. Int J Cardiol 1993;40:265–72.

38. Oberg B, Poulsen T. Obesity: an anesthetic challenge. Acta Anaesthesiol Scand 1996;40:191–200.

39. Mabie W, Ratts T, Ramanathan K, et al. Circulatory congestion in obese hypertensive women. A subset of pulmonary edema in pregnancy. Obstet Gynecol 1988; 72:553–8.

40. Elkus R, Popovich J. Respiratory physiology in pregnancy. Clin Chest Med 1992; 13:555–65.

41. Eng M, Butler J, Bonica JJ. Respiratory function in pregnant obese women. Am J Obstet Gynecol 1975;123:241–5.

42. Pelosi P, Croci M, Ravagnan L, et al. The effects of body mass on lung volumes, respiratory mechanics, and gas exchange during general anesthesia. Anesth Analg 1998;87:654–60.

43. Izci B, Riha RL, Martin SE, et al. The upper airway in pregnancy and pre-eclampsia. Am J Respir Crit Care Med 2003;167:137–40.

44. Pilkington S, Carli F, Dakin MJ, et al. Increase in Mallampati score during pregnancy. Br J Anaesth 1995;74:638–42.

45. Marik PE, Plante LA. Venous thromboembolic disease and pregnancy. N Engl J Med 2008;359:2025–33.

46. Heit JA, Kobbervig CE, James AH, et al. Trends in the incidence of venous thromboembolism during pregnancy or postpartum: a 30-year population-based study. Ann Intern Med 2005;143:697–706.

47. Burrow G. Thyroid function and hyperfunction during gestation. Endocr Rev 1993;14:194–202.

48. Glinoer D. The regulation of thyroid function in pregnancy: pathways of endocrine adaptation from physiology to pathology. Endocr Rev 1997;18:404–33.

49. Kissebah A, Bydelingum N, Murray R, et al. Relation of body height and fat distribution to metabolic complications of obesity. J Clin Endocrinol Metab 1982;54:254–60.

50. Catalano PM, Tyzbir ED, Wolfe RR, et al. Carbohydrate metabolism during pregnancy in control subjects and women with gestational diabetes. Am J Physiol 1993;264:E60–7.

51. O'Sullivan G, Scrutton M. NPO during labor: is there any scientific validation? Anesthesiol Clin North America 2003;21:87–98.
52. Baron TH, Ramirez B, Richter JE. Gastrointestinal motility disorders during pregnancy. Ann Intern Med 1993;118:366–75.
53. Baskett TF, Sternadel J. Maternal intensive care and near-miss mortality in obstetrics. Br J Obstet Gynaecol 1998;105:981–4.
54. Kilpatrick SJ, Matthay MA. Obstetric patients requiring critical care. A five-year review. Chest 1992;101:1407–12.
55. Lapinsky SE, Kruczynski K, Slutsky AS. Critical care in the pregnant patient. Am J Respir Crit Care Med 1995;152:427–55.
56. The American College of Obstetricians and Gynecologists (ACOG) and The American College of Allergy, Asthma and Immunology (ACAAI). The use of newer asthma and allergy medications during pregnancy. Ann Allergy Asthma Immunol 2000;84:475–80.
57. Stenius-Aarniala BS, Hedman J, Teramo KA. Acute asthma during pregnancy. Thorax 1996;51:411–4.
58. Wendel PJ, Ramin SM, Barnett-Hamm C, et al. Asthma treatment in pregnancy: a randomized controlled study. Am J Obstet Gynecol 1996;175:150–4.
59. Gonik B. Intensive care monitoring of the critically ill pregnant patient. In: Creasy RK, Resnik R, editors. Maternal-fetal medicine. Philadelphia: W.B. Saunders; 1999. p. 895–920.
60. Langeron O, Amour J, Vivien B, et al. Clinical review: management of difficult airways. Crit Care 2006;10:243–7.
61. Baraka AS, Taha SK, Aouad MT, et al. Preoxygenation: comparison of maximal breathing and tidal volume techniques. Anesthesiology 1999;91:612–6.
62. Lewin SB, Cheek TG, Deutschman CS. Airway management in the obstetric patient. Crit Care Clin 2000;16:505–13.
63. Hawthorne L, Wilson R, Lyons G, et al. Failed intubation revisited: a 17-yr experience in a teaching maternity unit. Br J Anaesth 1996;76:680–4.
64. Hawkins JL. Anesthesia-related maternal mortality. Clin Obstet Gynecol 2003;46:679–87.
65. Acute Respiratory Distress Syndrome Network. Ventilation with lower tidal volumes as compared with traditional tidal volumes for acute lung injury and the acute respiratory distress syndrome. N Engl J Med 2000;342:1301–8.
66. Tomlinson MW, Caruthers TJ, Whitty JE, et al. Does delivery improve maternal condition in the respiratory-compromised gravida? Obstet Gynecol 1998;91:108–11.
67. Hollmen AI, Jouppila R, Jouppila P. Regional anaesthesia and uterine blood flow. Ann Chir Gynaecol 1984;73:149–52.
68. Cooper DW, Carpenter M, Mowbray P, et al. Fetal and maternal effects of phenylephrine and ephedrine during spinal anesthesia for cesarean delivery. Anesthesiology 2002;97:1582–90.
69. Lee A, Ngan Kee WD, Gin T. A quantitative, systematic review of randomized controlled trials of ephedrine versus phenylephrine for the management of hypotension during spinal anesthesia for cesarean delivery. Anesth Analg 2002;94:920–6.
70. Merlino G, Scaglione R, Paterna S, et al. Lymphocyte beta-adrenergic receptors in young subjects with peripheral or central obesity: relationship with central haemodynamics and left ventricular function. Eur Heart J 1994;15:786–92.
71. Lowe SA. Diagnostic radiography in pregnancy: risks and reality. Aust N Z J Obstet Gynaecol 2004;44:191–6.

72. Vasquez DN, Estenssoro E, Canales H, et al. Clinical characteristics and outcomes of obstetric patients requiring ICU admission. Chest 2007;131:718–24.
73. Lewinsohn G, Herman A, Leonov Y, et al. Critically ill obstetrical patients: outcome and predictability. Crit Care Med 1994;22:1412–4.
74. Karnard D, Lapsia V, Krishnan A, et al. Prognostic factors in obstetric patients admitted to an Indian intensive care unit. Crit Care Med 2004;32:1294–9.
75. Chang-hun Tang L, Chi-wai Kwok A. Critical care in obstetrical patients: an eight-year review. Chin Med J 1997;110:936–41.
76. Gilbert TT, Smulian JC, Martin AA, et al. Obstetric admissions to the intensive care unit: outcomes and severity of illness. Obstet Gynecol 2003;102:897–903.
77. Bhagwanjee S, Paruk F, Moddley J, et al. Intensive care unit morbidity and mortality from preeclampsia: an evaluation of the acute physiology and chronic health evaluation ii score and the Glasgow coma scale score. Crit Care Med 2000;28:120–4.
78. Geller SE, Rosenberg D, Cox S, et al. A scoring system identified near-miss maternal morbidity during pregnancy. J Clin Epidemiol 2004;57:716–20.
79. Keirse MJ. Endogenous prostaglandins in human parturition. In: Keirse MJ, Anderson AB, Bennebroek GJ, editors. Human parturition. Leiden (Netherland): Leiden University Press; 1979. p. 101.
80. Turnbull AC. The endocrine control of labour. In: Turnbull AC, Chamberlain G, editors. Obstetrics. London: Churchill Livingston; 1989. p. 189.
81. Haluska GJ, Cook MJ, Novy MJ. Inhibition and augmentations of progesterone production during pregnancy: effects on parturition in rhesus monkeys. Am L Obstet Gynecol 1997;176:682–91.
82. Fuchs AR. The role of oxytocin in parturition. In: Huszar G, editor. The Physiology and biochemistry of the uterus in pregnancy and labour. 9th edition. Boca Raton (FL): CRC Press; 1986. p. 163.
83. Zeeman GG, Khan-Dawoos FS, Dawoosd MY. Oxytocin and its receptor in pregnancy and parturition: current concepts and clinical implications. Obstet Gynecol 1997;889:873.
84. Campbell EA, Linton E, Wolfe CD, et al. Plasma corticotrophin-releasing hormone concentrations during pregnancy and parturition. J Clin Endocrinol Metab 1987;64:1054.
85. Maclennan AH, Niclson R, Green RC. Serum relaxin in pregnancy. Lancet 1986;2:241.
86. Dudley DJ. Preterm labor: an intra-uterine inflammatory response syndrome? J Reprod Immunol 1997;36:93.
87. Cunningham GF, Leveno KJ, Bloom SL. Williams obstetrics. 23rd edition. New York: McGraw Hill Professional; 2009.
88. Whitty RJ, Maxwell CV, Carvalho JC. Complications of neuraxial anesthesia in an extreme morbidly obese patient for cesarean section. Int J Obstet Anesth 2007;16:139–44.
89. Hamilton CL, Riley ET, Cohen SE. Changes in their position of epidural catheters associated with patient movement. Anesthesiology 1997;86:778–84.
90. Douglas MJ, Flanagan MK, McMortland GH. Anesthetic management of a complex morbidly obese parturient. Can J Anaesth 1191;38;900-3
91. ACOG. Practice Bulletin. Clinical management guidelines for obstetrician-gynecologist. Number 17, June 2000.
92. Sanchez-Ramos L, Kaunitz AM, Delke I. Labor induction with 25 microg versus 50 microg intravaginal misoprostol: a systematic review. Obstet Gynecol 2002;99:145–51.

93. Calder AA, Loughney AD, Weir CJ, et al. Induction of labour in nulliparous women; a UK, multicentre, open-label study of intravaginal misoprostol in comparison with dinoprostone. BJOG 2008;115:1279–88.
94. Le Roux PA, Olarogun JO, Penny J, et al. Oral and vaginal misoprostol compared with dinoprostone for induction of labour: a randomized controlled trial. Obstet Gynecol 2002;99:201.
95. de Groot AN, van Dongen PW, Vree TB, et al. Ergot and alkaloids. Current status and review of clinical pharmacology and therapeutic use compared with other oxytocins. Obstetrics and gynecology. Drugs 1998;56(4):523–35.
96. American College of Obstetricians and Gynecologist, American College of Obstetricians and Gynecologists Practice Bulletin. Operative vaginal delivery. Washington, DC: American College of Obstetricians and Gynecologists; 2000.
97. Maughan KL, Heim SW. Preventing postpartum hemorrhage: managing the third stage of labor. Am Fam Physician 2006;73(6):1025–8.

Afterword
Sensitivity in Caring for the Obese Patient

Caring for the obese patient requires sensitivity by health care professionals not only to the patient but also to the family members. Our personal opinions need to be set aside when providing care. Sensitivity training can be an eye-opening experience for health care workers as some do not realize they have such a bias to obesity. In several studies, physicians and nursing personnel were found to have weight bias and overall negative feelings about obese patients.[1] This negative bias has an impact on the obese patient both psychologically and physically.[2] Being sensitive to the obese patient and their families instills confidence and reassurance in their health care providers.[3]

There are many things to consider when caring for the obese patient. Providing obese patients with appropriate-sized gowns can make the patient feel more confident to get out of bed and ambulate. Having appropriate lifts, walkers, beds, and commodes will also enable the obese patient to participate more in their care as they will not be afraid their size may hurt someone. Many obese patients are afraid to ask for assistance or even seek health care due to the stigma associated with obesity. Having waiting room chairs without arms or benches may provide seating comfort for those visitors who are obese.[3] Regardless of their size as a patient, they deserve to be treated with respect, dignity, and sensitivity.

Michele Chamberlain, BSN, RN, CBN
Bariatric Surgery Department
Geisinger Medical Center
100 North Academy Avenue
Danville, PA 17822, USA

E-mail address:
mkchamberlain@geisinger.edu

REFERENCES

1. Schwartz MB, Chambliss HO, Brownell KD, et al. Weight bias among health professionals specializing in obesity. Obes Res 2003;11:1033–9.
2. Brown I. Nurses' attitudes towards adult patients who are obese: literature review. J Adv Nurs 2006;53:221–32.
3. Puhl R. The stigma of obesity: a review and update. Obesity (Silver Spring) 2009; 17(5):941–64.

Index

Note: Page numbers of article titles are in **boldface** type.

Crit Care Clin 26 (2010) 735–741
doi:10.1016/S0749-0704(10)00079-5
0749-0704/10/$ – see front matter © 2010 Elsevier Inc. All rights reserved.

criticalcare.theclinics.com

1. Publication Title	2. Publication Number	3. Filing Date
Critical Care Clinics	0 0 0 - 7 0 8	9/15/10

4. Issue Frequency	5. Number of Issues Published Annually	6. Annual Subscription Price
Jan, Apr, Jul, Oct	4	$167.00

7. Complete Mailing Address of Known Office of Publication (Not printer) (Street, city, county, state, and ZIP+4®)

Elsevier Inc.
360 Park Avenue South
New York, NY 10010-1710

Contact Person
Stephen Bushing
Telephone (Include area code)
215-239-3688

8. Complete Mailing Address of Headquarters or General Business Office of Publisher (Not printer)

Elsevier Inc., 360 Park Avenue South, New York, NY 10010-1710

9. Full Names and Complete Mailing Addresses of Publisher, Editor, and Managing Editor (Do not leave blank)

Publisher (Name and complete mailing address)

Kim Murphy, Elsevier, Inc., 1600 John F. Kennedy Blvd. Suite 1800, Philadelphia, PA 19103-2899

Editor (Name and complete mailing address)

Patrick Manley, Elsevier, Inc., 1600 John F. Kennedy Blvd. Suite 1800, Philadelphia, PA 19103-2899

Managing Editor (Name and complete mailing address)

Catherine Bewick, Elsevier, Inc., 1600 John F. Kennedy Blvd. Suite 1800, Philadelphia, PA 19103-2899

10. Owner (Do not leave blank. If the publication is owned by a corporation, give the name and address of the corporation immediately followed by the names and addresses of all stockholders owning or holding 1 percent or more of the total amount of stock. If not owned by a corporation, give the names and addresses of the individual owners. If owned by a partnership or other unincorporated firm, give its name and address as well as those of each individual owner. If the publication is published by a nonprofit organization, give its name and address.)

Full Name	Complete Mailing Address
Wholly owned subsidiary of	4520 East-West Highway
Reed/Elsevier, US holdings	Bethesda, MD 20814

11. Known Bondholders, Mortgagees, and Other Security Holders Owning or Holding 1 Percent or More of Total Amount of Bonds, Mortgages, or Other Securities. If none, check box ☐ None

Full Name	Complete Mailing Address
N/A	

12. Tax Status (For completion by nonprofit organizations authorized to mail at nonprofit rates) (Check one)
The purpose, function, and nonprofit status of this organization and the exempt status for federal income tax purposes:
☐ Has Not Changed During Preceding 12 Months
☐ Has Changed During Preceding 12 Months (Publisher must submit explanation of change with this statement)

PS Form 3526, September 2007 (Page 1 of 3 (Instructions Page 3)) PSN 7530-01-000-9931 PRIVACY NOTICE: See our Privacy policy in www.usps.com

---

13. Publication Title	14. Issue Date for Circulation Data Below
Critical Care Clinics	July 2010

15. Extent and Nature of Circulation			Average No. Copies Each Issue During Preceding 12 Months	No. Copies of Single Issue Published Nearest to Filing Date
a. Total Number of Copies (Net press run)			1834	1700
b. Paid Circulation (By Mail and Outside the Mail)	(1)	Mailed Outside-County Paid Subscriptions Stated on PS Form 3541. (Include paid distribution above nominal rate, advertiser's proof copies, and exchange copies)	858	853
	(2)	Mailed In-County Paid Subscriptions Stated on PS Form 3541 (Include paid distribution above nominal rate, advertiser's proof copies, and exchange copies)		
	(3)	Paid Distribution Outside the Mails Including Sales Through Dealers and Carriers, Street Vendors, Counter Sales, and Other Paid Distribution Outside USPS®	366	358
	(4)	Paid Distribution by Other Classes Mailed Through the USPS (e.g. First-Class Mail®)		
c. Total Paid Distribution (Sum of 15b (1), (2), (3), and (4))			1224	1211
d. Free or Nominal Rate Distribution (By Mail and Outside the Mail)	(1)	Free or Nominal Rate Outside-County Copies Included on PS Form 3541	96	85
	(2)	Free or Nominal Rate In-County Copies Included on PS Form 3541		
	(3)	Free or Nominal Rate Copies Mailed at Other Classes Through the USPS (e.g. First-Class Mail)		
	(4)	Free or Nominal Rate Distribution Outside the Mail (Carriers or other means)		
e. Total Free or Nominal Rate Distribution (Sum of 15d (1), (2), (3) and (4))			96	85
f. Total Distribution (Sum of 15c and 15e)			1320	1296
g. Copies not Distributed (See instructions to publishers #4 (page #3))			514	404
h. Total (Sum of 15f and g)			1834	1700
i. Percent Paid (15c divided by 15f times 100)			92.73%	93.44%

16. Publication of Statement of Ownership
☐ If the publication is a general publication, publication of this statement is required. Will be printed in the October 2010 issue of this publication.   ☐ Publication not required.

17. Signature and Title of Editor, Publisher, Business Manager, or Owner

Stephen R. Bushing

Stephen R. Bushing – Fulfillment/Inventory Specialist

Date
September 15, 2010

I certify that all information furnished on this form is true and complete. I understand that anyone who furnishes false or misleading information on this form or who omits material or information requested on the form may be subject to criminal sanctions (including fines and imprisonment) and/or civil sanctions (including civil penalties).

PS Form 3526, September 2007 (Page 2 of 3)

Moving?

Make sure your subscription moves with you!

To notify us of your new address, find your **Clinics Account Number** (located on your mailing label above your name), and contact customer service at:

Email: journalscustomerservice-usa@elsevier.com

800-654-2452 (subscribers in the U.S. & Canada)
314-447-8871 (subscribers outside of the U.S. & Canada)

Fax number: 314-447-8029

Elsevier Health Sciences Division
Subscription Customer Service
3251 Riverport Lane
Maryland Heights, MO 63043

*To ensure uninterrupted delivery of your subscription, please notify us at least 4 weeks in advance of move.

Printed and bound by CPI Group (UK) Ltd, Croydon, CR0 4YY

03/10/2024

01040462-0013